CONTENTS

GW00726916

Acknowledgements

My thanks go to Linda Dodimead, Senior Paediatric Dietician at the Whittington Hospital, London, for her help in creating the 'Food Diary', and to colleagues, such as Gillie Kennedy, who so willingly share their experience, enabling the professions to grow.

Foreword

While speech and language therapists have been involved with the management of feeding problems in children for some considerable time, it is only comparatively recently that the focus of their input has included babies.

The legacy of modern technology is a cohort of infants who survive in spite of being born prematurely – in some cases up to 18 weeks early – and who can present with complex needs in relation to their feeding. It is fast being recognized by other professionals who care for these infants that feeding is often the persisting problem which prevents discharge from the costly neonatal unit. Consequently referrals of such babies are increasing, with demand often challenging the present resources, both of establishment and of therapists' knowledge-base. Similarly, speech and language therapists who work as part of child development teams are expected to continue the care of these often medically fragile infants in the community without immediate access to medical or nursing colleagues, unlike their more fortunate acute unit counterparts.

Arlene McCurtin's book is based upon practical experience of being in such a situation and in addition to this she has worked with toddlers and young children who have had continuing difficulties with eating and/or drinking. She is acutely aware of the need to identify feeding difficulties and associated problems, such as reflux, early on in the infant's development in order to allay the potential development of persistent so-called 'behavioural' eating and drinking issues.

This book will be a useful resource for those therapists who work in any setting with infants or young children presenting with feeding difficulties.

Gillian Kennedy, Principal Speech & Language Therapist, The Middlesex and University College Hospitals, UK
April 1997

About the Author

Since qualifying as a speech and language therapist in 1985 Arlene McCurtin has worked in Canada, England and Ireland predominantly with children with special needs. This has fostered a special interest in paediatric feeding difficulties and, while working with Camden and Islington Health Authority in London, Arlene was responsible for setting up a multidisciplinary feeding clinic.

In her current position as Principal Speech and Language Therapist at the Central Remedial Clinic, Dublin, the emphasis on feeding problems continues, most especially with children with physical and multiple disabilities from a month old but also, more recently, to adults with physical disabilities.

Arlene obtained her undergraduate degree at Trinity College, Dublin in 1985 and an MSc at City University, London in 1994.

INTRODUCTION

In recent years there has been a growing recognition of, interest in and emphasis on paediatric feeding disorders and the significance of feeding difficulties for feeders, children and professionals. This can be attributed to several factors: the natural development of the appropriate professions; the emphasis on multidisciplinary work; the growing understanding of and focus on developmental problems; the ability to assess and treat at earlier and more severe levels of disability; the importance of feeding to nutrition and general development; and the increasing numbers of children surviving, as a result of medical and technological advances, at earlier gestational levels, and with more profound and multiple problems.

This manual has been written in response to the general need to have practical and accessible assessment and therapy tools available in a busy clinic. Its style is intentionally problem-led and pragmatic to meet this objective, with applications for the range of professionals working with feeding disorders, such as speech and language therapists, occupational therapists and nurses.

Photocopying

Checklists and assessments are intended to serve a functional purpose and therefore can be photocopied by the purchaser of this manual for use with individual children.

Warning

The clinician should *stop and think* before using guidelines, and consider their relevance, safety and appropriateness with regard to the individual child. The guidelines, of necessity, are general in nature and the clinician must always consider the suitability of guidelines when thinking about applying them to individual children. This is especially relevant in children with feeding disorders, as the very nature of the feeding process, combined with the child's individual problems, means that great care must be taken when applying therapy techniques. The clinician must take responsibility for the selection and use of guidelines.

Editor's note

Please note that 'he' is used to refer to the child and 'she' to the therapist for the sake of clarity alone.

The oral, nasal and pharyngeal areas

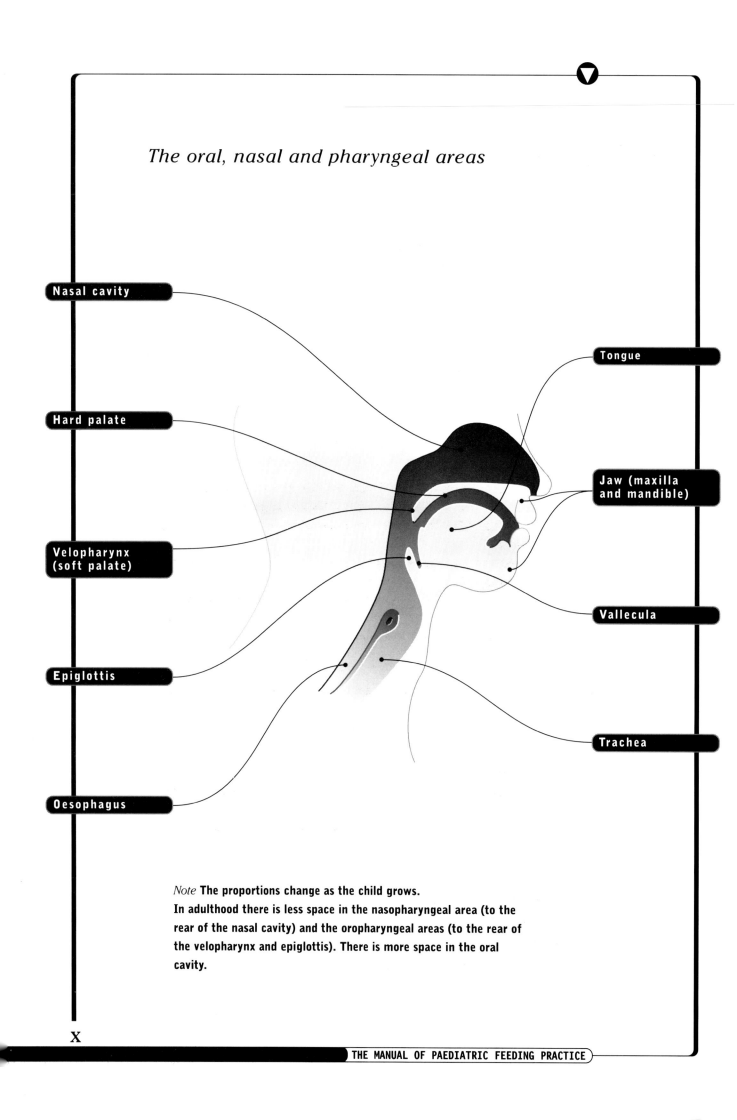

Nasal cavity

Hard palate

Velopharynx (soft palate)

Epiglottis

Oesophagus

Tongue

Jaw (maxilla and mandible)

Vallecula

Trachea

Note **The proportions change as the child grows.**
In adulthood there is less space in the nasopharyngeal area (to the rear of the nasal cavity) and the oropharyngeal areas (to the rear of the velopharynx and epiglottis). There is more space in the oral cavity.

ASSESSMENT GUIDELINES

1 ··· **Get information from other disciplines.** A multidisciplinary approach to feeding problems will enable the feeding difficulty to be dealt with in a more efficient manner, ensure support for each professional's goals and minimize confusion for the parents. Professionals involved in feeding problems include health visitors, paediatric dieticians, paediatric occupational therapists, specialist speech and language therapists, paediatric physiotherapists, radiologists, paediatric surgeons and paediatricians.

2 ··· **Read the child's medical history** or consult relevant professionals to familiarize yourself with the child's history and conditions which may influence the feeding process and treatment goals.

3 ··· Ask the feeder to fill in the photocopiable **'Food Diary'** (page 71) before the initial session. This has a number of advantages:

▼ It gives the feeder an opportunity to think about the particular feeding difficulties and the child's skills and specific problem areas;
▼ It will ensure that the parent has information on hand for the first session;
▼ It hands some of the responsibility over to the parent for helping to solve problems and treat the feeding difficulty;
▼ It empowers parents by involving them in the therapy process;
▼ It provides preliminary immediate information for the professional;
▼ It provides an overview of the parent's understanding and construction of the child's feeding skills and the feeding process.

4 ··· Where appropriate, **encourage the parents to observe and assess jointly** with the therapist using the assessment checklist if appropriate, or through general discussion and highlighting of specific areas. This will:

▼ help feeder observation skills;
▼ encourage the feeder's responsibility in the process of change and decision making;
▼ help in the development of a partnership with the clinician;
▼ empower the feeder.

5 ··· **Identify the problem area/s through a combined process of assessment and diagnostic therapy.** This can be achieved in a number of ways:

▼ familiarization with the medical history and conditions;
▼ direct assessment;
▼ observation;

1

▼ discussion with the main feeder;
▼ probing and trials;
▼ monitoring the child's state and responses to changes in the feeding process.

6 ··· **Arrange a home visit** if at all possible. This gives the therapist an opportunity to observe a number of important areas:

▼ the home set-up at feeding time;
▼ feeding equipment and utensils;
▼ family resources;
▼ family patterns of eating;
▼ family interactions.

7 ··· Where appropriate, **make use of technologies and resources** such as barium swallow and videofluoroscopy. If these facilities are not available in the child's immediate area, try to make use of them where they are available and, if possible, build links to make them more readily available to feeding therapists and children with feeding difficulties.

Use of technology can fulfil a number of important functions:

▼ diagnosis of the presence and extent of specific anatomical and functional problems;
▼ evaluation of the feeding process as a whole;
▼ diagnosis of specific conditions which may significantly affect feeding and progress, such as aspiration and reflux;
▼ feeder understanding of what is happening during feeding and the causal or contributory factors;
▼ confidence and direction in treatment goals;
▼ increase the understanding of the problem and therefore the ability to make changes.

8 ··· **Provide clear written recommendations and guidelines** to feeders and other professionals after the assessment is complete. This should include identification of specific problem areas, and treatment suggestions.

9 ··· **Grade recommendations.** Providing too much information and too many recommendations can confuse a feeder and reduce the effectiveness of the recommendations. When making recommendations, consider:

▼ the immediate and important problems areas;
▼ which recommendation will have a positive effect on feeding;
▼ feeder readiness and capacity for absorbing information and achieving carry-over.

10 ·· As feeding behaviours can be difficult to evaluate, **do not expect definite and immediate assessment results.** This is especially important with regard to the following:

▼ **invisible processes such as reflux and aspiration;**

▼ **oral functions and patterns such as swallowing and tongue movements (lips closure during feeding generally inhibits exact observation of this);**

▼ **the etiology, as it can prove difficult to discriminate between behaviour, communication or oro-motor acts.**

GRADING AND ASSESSMENT

The feeding checklist on the following pages is intended to be a general guide about what to observe, evaluate and chart during the feeding assessment session. For a more detailed analysis of suspected problems, see the relevant sections. For example, to assess for possible aspiration, see the section entitled 'Aspiration'.

The summary chart at the end of the assessment provides an opportunity to summarize and quantify identified problem areas. Quantification is useful for determining the severity of a problem, for conveying this information to others and for measuring progress. However, quantification of feeding problems is open to subjectivity and, to lessen the impact of this, the clinician making the quantification for the individual child should be consistent. Where teams are concerned, they need to agree on what constitutes each level. Specific grading for specific problems is available in relevant sections of this book. For example, to grade suck function, see 'Co-ordination of the suck – swallow – breathe pattern'. The following are general guidelines.

Severity	Grades	Characteristics
NORMAL	GRADE 0	*No problem present which affects feeding*
MILD	GRADE 1	*Slightly affects feeding*
MODERATE	GRADE 2	*Affects success of tube/oral feeding but does not disrupt process significantly*
SEVERE	GRADE 3	*Significantly affects oral feeding/ moderately affects success of tube feeding*
PROFOUND	GRADE 4	*Prevents oral feeding/significantly affects success of tube feeding*

3

FEEDING ASSESSMENT CHECKLIST

NAME	DATE
CHRONOLOGICAL AGE	**CORRECTED/DEVELOPMENTAL AGE**

Part 1: *Feeder Interview*

AREA 1 MEDICAL & HISTORY	NOTES
Pregnancy and birth • Prenatal history • Gestational age • Birth history • Post natal history	
Current medical diagnoses, conditions and monitoring	
Surgical interventions	
Relevant family history	
Use of medications • Names • Reasons for use • Response to use	
Feeding history and experiences • Tube feeding • Attempts at oral feeding • Weight gain	
Professionals involved in feeding management	
Modifications made to feeding and utensils	

4

THE MANUAL OF PAEDIATRIC FEEDING PRACTICE

Part 2: *Observations and Probes*

AREA 2 MOTOR	NOTES
Motor skills • General body tone (hypotonia/hypertonia) • Limiting conditions or patterns	
Positioning • Child during feeding • Feeder during feeding • Child after feeding	
Self-feeding skills	

AREA 3 EQUIPMENT	NOTES
Seating equipment	
Utensils used	

AREA 4 NUTRITIONAL	NOTES
Method of feeding • Oral • Oro/nasogastric tube • Gastrostomy • Combined feeding	
Amount of intake • Amount given per meal • Amount taken, less spillage • Quantities per method • Note variable intake	
Food consistencies • Offered • Accepted • Amount per consistency • Main consistency used	
Range of tastes • Tastes offered • Tastes accepted • Main flavours used • Child's preferred taste	
Weight • Current weight and centile • Use of supplements	

AREA 5 ORO-MOTOR	NOTES
Anatomical structures • Lips • Tongue • Cheeks • Jaw • Hard palate • Soft palate • Teeth • Other	
Limiting patterns and effects • Lips • Tongue • Cheeks • Jaw • Hard palate • Soft palate • Teeth • Other	
Sucking • Presence of non-nutritive suck • Presence of nutritive suck • Strength of suck • Initiation of suck • Co-ordination of suck – swallow – breathe pattern	
Swallowing • Presence of swallowing reflex • Timing of swallow • Co-ordination of suck – swallow – breathe pattern	
Sensation • Normal • Hypersensitivity present • Hyposensitivity present • Areas affected	
Speech development • Vowels • Consonants • Nasality	
Oral hygiene	

THE MANUAL OF PAEDIATRIC FEEDING PRACTICE

AREA 6 ENVIRONMENTAL	NOTES
Feeder • Main feeder • Other feeders • State • Expectations • Communication cues used • Attitudes to food • Parental health	
Feeding routine • Length of feeds • Number of feeds • Times of feeds • Location(s) of feeds	
Environmental stimuli • Visual • Auditory • Adults/peers present	
Sociocultural factors • which may affect feeding	

AREA 7 BEHAVIOUR	NOTES
Behaviour and mood • Before feeding • During feeding • After feeding	
Responses • To initiation of feeding • To changes in feeding	
Child's communication modes and signals during feeding • Communication mode(s) • Specific acts used • Interaction with peers	

AREA 8 ASSOCIATED CONDITIONS	NOTES
Indications of reflux and/or aspiration	
Respiratory • Evidence of compromise	
Endurance • Evidence of bradycardia/ tachycardia	

Part 3: *Summary Observations*

AREA	SPECIFIC DIFFICULTIES PRESENT	GRADE
MEDICAL & HISTORY		
MOTOR		
EQUIPMENT		
NUTRITIONAL		
ORO–MOTOR		
ENVIRONMENTAL		
BEHAVIOUR		
ASSOCIATED CONDITIONS		

TREATMENT GUIDELINES

1 ··· **Familiarize yourself with the child's medical history and condition.**

2 ··· **Liaise with other professionals** involved in treatment of the feeding difficulties. This will ensure:

- ▼ **less confusion for parents;**
- ▼ **a more complete treatment plan;**
- ▼ **an awareness of the priorities of other professionals.**

3 ··· Remember that **each child is an individual.** This has significant implications because of the child's:

- ▼ **response to therapy in general;**
- ▼ **response to specific strategies;**
- ▼ **medical condition;**
- ▼ **home and school environments.**

4 ··· Try to **move at the child's pace.**

5 ··· **Implement changes gradually.** Graded changes in all areas (eg. consistency) have an increased chance of success. Do not set changes in motion too quickly or make changes too extreme. This is particularly important when treating children with hypersensitivity or medical conditions which can dramatically affect their ability to adapt to changes, such as children with reduced endurance, respiratory compromise and poor neurological states.

6 ··· **Correct positioning of the child has a significant effect on the potential for effective treatment.** Inappropriate positioning can seriously reduce the effects of treatment goals and strategies.

7 ··· **Feeding time should be limited to a maximum of between 20 and 30 minutes.** This ensures that the child is able to cope with the process and does not tire too quickly, particularly in cases of unstable neurological states, reduced endurance and significant oro-motor dysfunction. It also, therefore, reduces the possibility of aversive behavioural acts occurring or increasing in frequency.

8 ··· **Always monitor the child's responses to feeding** and changes in feeding, particularly in cases of reduced endurance, respiratory compromise and oro-motor dysfunction, and with preterm babies.

9 ··· With older children, **learn their communication signals,** which mode they are made in, and whether they indicate negative or positive feelings.

9

10 ·· **Have consistent feeders.** This is particularly important when the child is in settings such as a hospital, nursery or school.

11 ·· **Ensure consistent practice** and follow-through of recommendations. Establish a routine. If there are difficulties with carrying out particular recommendations, evaluate how the recommendations or environment can be adapted. If the home environment is not proving conducive to feeding development, explore the potential for using different environments, such as nurseries.

12 ·· **Explore the feeder's** interaction, mind-set, aims and ability to carry out suggestions.

13 ·· Where children need to concentrate on the feeding process, reduce or **minimize environmental distractions** which may affect their concentration on feeding. The feeding environment should be warm and relaxing. This is particularly relevant with children who have visual impairments, profound and multiple difficulties or unstable neurological states, and with premature babies.

14 ·· **Preparatory handling** is necessary with children who have increased or decreased tone and unstable neurological states. This will help to stabilize and prepare the child for feeding.

15 ·· Remember that **feeding therapy may be a long-term process** involving areas which take considerable effort and commitment from clinicians and carers to resolve. Remember also that there is no guarantee that problems can be resolved.

16 ·· **Use the 'Recommendations Sheet'** on the following page to provide written guidelines to the feeder. This will help understanding and carry-over of suggestions.

RECOMMENDATIONS SHEET

NAME	DATE

Always be aware of your child's ability to cope with new techniques by monitoring his/her breathing, comfort levels and adaptability.

TARGET AREA 1

FEEDING SUGGESTIONS

1 ...

2 ...

TARGET AREA 2

FEEDING SUGGESTIONS

1 ...

2 ...

TARGET AREA 3

FEEDING SUGGESTIONS

1 ...

2 ...

Overview

Aspiration is the inhalation of food material into the lungs. The stage at which aspiration occurs can be related to the predominant area of oral activity as described by Wolf and Glass (1992) – aspiration before the swallow, during the swallow and after the swallow.

Classification

Aspiration can be classified along three lines:

[1] · · · Swallowing stage at which it occurs, as outlined above.

[2] · · · Type of occurrence:

    a] chronic aspiration can refer to continually occurring aspiration;

    b] state-related aspiration can refer to aspiration which occurs when the child is respiratorially compromised, as with chest infections;

    c] fatigue aspiration occurs during the feeding session as the child tires;

    d] silent aspiration is not generally clinically evident, but can be picked up by radiological testing.

[3] · · · Severity of occurrence, as discussed in the grading section below, from normal to profound.

Causes and Contributory Factors

Aspiration *before* the swallow is primarily the result of abnormal tongue movements in the oral phase of swallowing, where bolus formation and retention is poor. Aspiration *during* the swallow is usually caused by reduced laryngeal elevation and closure. Aspiration *after* the swallow can be caused by reduced pharyngeal peristalsis or post nasal reflux and is usually secondary to inadequate clearance of food from the valleculae or pharyngeal area with residual liquids or solids remaining in the pharynx after the swallow (Wolf and Glass, 1992). Additionally, reflux, the return of stomach contents, can cause aspiration at this stage.

Neal (1995) has recently pointed out that methods used to provide respiratory support to premature babies, for example, continuous positive airway pressure (CPAP), may provoke aspiration in babies attempting to feed by sucking.

The clinician can usually detect at which stage aspiration is occurring by identifying the other problem areas and functions. However, radiological procedures, such as videofluoroscopy, barium swallow and chest X-ray, will be needed to confirm the presence of aspiration.

12

Grading and assessment

It is difficult to determine for certain without the aid of radiological techniques whether aspiration is a factor in the feeding process. However, there are clinical indications which can point to the presence of aspiration and therefore aid in the decision-making process for referral to radiology and treatment. The checklist in this section, based in part on characteristics identified by Wolf and Glass (1992), will aid the clinician in determining the presence of aspiration.

The presence of a few signs alone may not necessarily indicate that aspiration is present, but the possibility should always be considered because of the consequences for the feeding process, the impact on the child's attitude towards feeding and potential medical complications (such as chest infections or pneumonia).

It can also be hard to clarify what constitutes significant aspiration. Determining the severity can be done according to the clinical signs evident (see the 'Clinical Indications of Aspiration Checklist'); the impact of aspiration on the feeding process; the impact on the child's respiratory status; and evidence from radiological techniques.

The terms 'mild', 'moderate', 'severe' and 'profound' can be used to identify the extent of the problems, but to evaluate progress and the effect of changes made during therapy and medical management, aspiration can be graded as outlined below. For grading to be useful, the same clinician should grade the severity over time and, where teams are involved, the team should agree on the grading system used. Guidelines for this process are shown on the following page.

Severity	Grades	Characteristics
NORMAL	**GRADE 0 ASPIRATION**	• *No aspiration present* • *No clinical signs evident* • *No aspiration evident on radiology techniques*
MILD	**GRADE 1 ASPIRATION**	• *One or two clinical signs evident but only occurring infrequently and not affecting feeding process* • *No or insignificant aspiration evident from radiological techniques*
MODERATE	**GRADE 2 ASPIRATION**	• *More than two clinical signs evident in a number of areas* • *Child needs time to recover but feeding can continue with care* • *Occasional chest infections* • *Aspiration observed from radiological techniques, but occasional rather than frequent*
SEVERE	**GRADE 3 ASPIRATION**	• *Multiple clinical signs observed* • *Significant disruption of the feeding process and its effectiveness, with child spending at least as much time recovering as feeding.* • *Frequent chest infections* • *Easily evident and frequent on radiological techniques*
PROFOUND	**GRADE 4 ASPIRATION**	• *Multiple clinical signs observed* • *Oral feeding contraindicated* • *Constant chest infections, bouts of pneumonia* • *Aspiration easily evident and consistent on radiological techniques*

CLINICAL INDICATIONS OF ASPIRATION CHECKLIST

NAME	DATE

Part 1: *Clinical Observations*

AREA	PRESENT	ABSENT
RESPIRATORY • Recurrent chest infections • Recurrent bouts of pneumonia • Respiratory compromise or failure (apnoea, cyanotic attacks) • Wheezing • 'Gurgly' sounds		
ORO-MOTOR • Difficulties with co-ordinating the suck – swallow – breathe pattern • Delayed swallow reflex • Absent swallow • Reduced, unco-ordinated or other abnormal tongue movements • Reduced, poorly co-ordinated or other abnormal soft palate elevation		
MEDICAL CONDITIONS • Reduced endurance: does child get sleepy/finish feeding early? • Bradycardia (slow heart rate) – (unless the child is on a monitor, this sign can be difficult to evaluate) • Excess mucus production/ secretions (which may be present as the result of increased toxins caused by allergies or aspiration)		
ASSOCIATED CONDITIONS • Presence of reflux • Acute or recurrent coughing or choking • Loud attempts at throat clearance • Orofacial hypersensitivity		

Part 2: *Summary Observations*

QUESTION	ANSWER
• Is it probable that aspiration is present? • Is aspiration likely to be Grade 0, 1, 2, 3 or 4 in its effect on feeding and respiration? • Is respiration chronic, state-related, fatigue-related or silent (not clinically evident) in nature? • At which part of the swallowing phase (before, during or after) does aspiration occur? • Is referral to radiology warranted?	

Therapy guidelines

1 ··· **Refer for videofluoroscopy, barium swallow and chest X-ray** to determine the presence and extent of aspiration and reflux, and the factors which may be contributing to their presence.

2 ··· **Check medical stability** by consulting relevant medical personnel and medical history.

3 ··· **Always monitor the child's signals** to see how he is coping with the feeding process. Understanding and observing the child's signals and behaviour will help in anticipating and relieving aspiration.

4 ··· **Focus on the primary difficulty** by analyzing at which stage aspiration is occurring. This will help to identify the main problem area, such as co-ordination of the suck – swallow – breathe pattern, a delayed swallow reflex or reduced soft palate elevation. See specific guidelines, eg. Co-ordination of sucking – swallowing – breathing.

5 ··· **Provide correct positioning during and after feeding.** Improved positioning will provide more stability and control, as well as specifically reducing the need for less laryngeal elevation.

▼ **Ensure head flexion or chin tucking.**
▼ **Determine the extent to which a child depends on neck hyperextension or tongue protrusion to maintain an airway.**
▼ **Consider a standing position (standing frame).**
▼ **Upright positioning should be maintained for at least half an hour after meals. Evans-Morris and Dunn-Klein (1987) recommended a 90 degree to 30 degree (flexed) position as the most effective to help decrease the effects of aspiration. This is particularly important where aspiration occurs as a result of residual food in the larynx. Experiment to find the most suitable position.**
▼ **See 'Positioning' guidelines (pages 82–83).**
▼ **Consult the child's paediatric physiotherapist or occupational therapist.**

6 ··· **Use utensils which will help reduce aspiration.** Use an angle-necked bottle or a bottle held at an angle when feeding. This is important to ensure flexion is maintained. With cup drinking, flexion can be a problem. Try a cut-out cup (with a U-shaped indentation in the rim) in the initial stages. Alternatively, try straw drinking as a transitional stage from bottle to cup.

7 ··· When introducing oral feeding, or where reduced endurance or respiratory compromise is present, Wolf and Glass (1992) recommend the **use of very small therapeutic feeds** – controlled and specified amounts – while maintaining primary nutrition via the tube.

16

This will help the child to have an oral focus, and will assist work on desensitization and grading the introduction of oral feeds. For children with profound aspiration this may not be appropriate.

8 ··· With oral feeding, **reduce the amount given at each feed and increase the number of feeds**. This should not be more frequent than every two hours and, as the amount given at each feed is gradually increased, the interval between feeds should also lengthen.

9 ··· Where aspiration occurs during the swallow, **provide cold stimulation** to the anterior faucal arches (tonsillar area), to help activate a swallow appropriately.

▼ **Evans-Morris and Dunn-Klein (1987) recommend use, prior to feeding, of a cotton swab (dipped in water and then frozen), an ice stick (water frozen in a straw and the plastic partially removed) or a cold finger. When using a straw, remove only an inch of ice stick at a time, using the rest for gripping. Stimulate the faucal arches. (This technique should not be used with a child who has a tonic bite reflex.)**

▼ **Have small amounts of food ready after preparing the swallow. Observe for indications that a swallow has occurred.**

10 ·· **Stimulate a swallow directly** where aspiration during the swallow is a problem. This needs to be experimented with, and the child's coping and reactions should be noted:

▼ **Move the index finger down along the throat, from the chin to the adam's apple, in simulation of the swallowing process.**

▼ **Tap the tip of the tongue and the place on the hard palate (alveolar ridge) where the tongue should touch to initiate the swallow.**

11 ·· **Thicken the consistency of feeds**, as some children are less able to cope with and control thinner consistencies. Thicker foods will provide more sensory input, form a more cohesive bolus that does not seep, and move more slowly, allowing for more oral control. The increased weight of the food will also help prevent it from re-entering the oesophagus.

▼ **Use cereal to thicken liquids. The recommended formula is 1oz/ 28 ml of dry cereal to 2oz/56ml of milk (Winstock, 1994; Alexander, 1987).**

▼ **Use a cornflour and water mixture to thicken liquids.**

▼ **Use thicker liquids such as pineapple juice or milkshakes.**

▼ **Try puréed foods.**

▼ **Consult a paediatric dietician about commercial thickeners.**

17

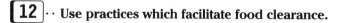

12 ·· Use practices which facilitate food clearance.

▼ Correct positioning as outlined previously.

▼ Thicken the consistency of foods, as outlined above.

▼ Establish a rhythm to feeding and swallowing which will help the child control and co-ordinate in an improved manner. Give verbal cues where appropriate: for example, 'Here comes the next spoon.'

▼ Encourage dry swallows by giving one or two boluses of thicker substances followed by several boluses of thinner liquids (Wolf and Glass, 1992). Maintaining chin tuck will minimize the effect of dry swallows.

▼ Allow the child to suck on a dummy during feeding, or after a single bolus.

13 ·· Avoid foods that contribute to the occurrence of aspiration or excess mucus production and which are less easily assimilated by the lungs. These include fats, milks, milk-based products, grains and some sweet foods (Wolf and Glass, 1992).

14 ·· Improve pharyngeal pressure and strengthen the vocal folds. Sometimes aspiration after the swallow is due to inadequate pressure, peristalsis and strength in moving the bolus through the pharynx into the oesophagus:

▼ Pushing activities can strengthen the vocal folds where they are appropriate and possible. Evans-Morris and Dunn-Klein (1987) recommend having the child push against the wall or the feeder's hands providing slight resistance. Having the child vocalize while doing so will help further. Make this activity as much fun as possible.

▼ Use a palatal training device, if possible, to improve velar function and velopharyngeal elevation. Consult the special needs dental officer.

15 ·· The use of suctioning equipment may be advisable where considerable aspiration is present. However, if the treatment is appropriately graded and the child's signals and state are monitored, this should be unnecessary.

16 ·· In cases of severe aspiration, considerably reduced endurance or significant respiratory compromise, **provide nutrition through non-oral means**. Eliminate oral feeding, but continue working on oro-motor desensitization and development.

Overview

Satter (1986) calls eating a 'sensitive barometer of emotional state' and clinicians working with children with feeding disorders may observe behavioural and communication acts, more at feeding time than at other times, which indicate the child's emotional state and coping behaviours.

Causes and Contributory Factors

Behaviours observed during feeding can function in a number of ways:

1 · · · They can be the child's method of communication.

2 · · · They can occur as a response to negative experiences such as reflux or a difficult feeding history.

3 · · · Some behaviours may in fact be reactions to changes that overload and disorganize a system that is not yet ready to cope with them.

4 · · · Observed behaviours may be the result of feeder–child interaction problems such as inappropriate feeding style or general management.

5 · · · Since children are sensitive to their feeder's moods and feelings (such as anxiety about feeding or nutritional issues), behaviours and communication acts may result in whole or in part from the child's reaction to the feeder's behaviour.

Normal Development

Reilly *et al* (1995) noted in their study that food refusal is common in the 12–18 month age range, as children are beginning to develop some independence in eating. Communication development is noted in detail in other texts. See the checklists in this section for help in the evaluation of communication and behaviours.

STRESS BEHAVIOURS CHECKLIST

NAME		DATE	
STRESS BEHAVIOURS	**PRESENT**	**ABSENT**	**SPECIFIC BEHAVIOUR**
STATE SIGNALS: subtle defence mechanism			
1 ··· Sudden changes, including becoming alert, drowsiness or disorganized sleepiness.			
2 ··· Non-verbal signals, such as facial grimaces or flaccidity, panicky or worried expressions, or tongue extensions.			
3 ··· General behaviours, such as irritability, fussing or strained crying.			
MOTOR SIGNALS: subtle defence mechanism			
1 ··· Hypertonic, tensing movements, such as limb extensions, arching, tongue extension, jerks or eye closing.			
2 ··· Hypotonic developments, such as flaccidity in any body part.			
3 ··· Tonal variability.			
AUTONOMIC SIGNALS: ultimate defence mechanism			
1 ··· Colour changes (to red or white) in the limbs, eyes, nails or mouth.			
2 ··· Changes in respiration: rate increase or decrease.			
3 ··· Changes in heart rate: bradycardia or tachycardia.			
4 ··· Pharyngeal/laryngeal activity such as gagging, choking, hiccoughs, vomiting.			

It can be difficult with children who have no refined communication system to interpret how they are handling feeding. When a child presents with an unstable neurological state, is premature or at an early developmental level, it is useful to look at non-intentional behaviours or signals, for the following reasons:

1 ··· This may help the clinician and feeder to understand the child's communication system.

2 ··· It is essential to monitor the child's coping system for safety reasons.

3 ··· It may reduce the potential for aversive behaviours developing.

4 ··· It aids perception of how the child is coping with changes made during feeding and helps the clinician and feeder grade changes appropriately.

5 ··· Feeding behaviour can be a sensitive indicator of a neonate's central nervous system integrity and of children with unstable neurological states.

The checklist on page 20 is based on Heidelise's (1986) identification of stress behaviours; the clinician notes whether a type of behaviour is present or absent, and identifies the specific behaviours.

COMMUNICATION BEHAVIOURS CHECKLIST

NAME		DATE	
TIME OF OBSERVATION	FROM		TO

What did the child do to communicate?	What mode was used?	What happened just before the communication?	What was the feeder's immediate response?

THE MANUAL OF PAEDIATRIC FEEDING PRACTICE

The communication behaviours checklist can be used to assess whether and to what extent the child communicates during feeding. This is a general checklist which can help to indicate exactly how the child communicates and the child's developmental level or abilities.

For best results, it is recommended that the feeder/clinician fill in this checklist either while the other is feeding the child or, preferably, while watching a videotape of the child feeding. This will help in a number of areas:

▼ **it promotes feeder participation;**
▼ **it helps feeder understanding and recognition of the child's signals;**
▼ **it helps the feeder to match the feeding process to the child and to grade changes appropriately. This is particularly important in children with an unstable neurological state, children with complex and multiple disabilities, and children with behavioural problems.**

In column 1, the specific act the child used is identified. (To analyse stress behaviours such as state-related and autonomic responses in more detail, see the 'Stress Behaviours Checklist', above.) Column 2 indicates the means of communication. Means or mode should be interpreted as the broad area of the communication act. Examples of modes are as follows:

STATE	• *Alerting (eg. to request food)* • *Crying (eg. to convey discomfort or hunger)* • *Sleepiness (eg. to indicate child's hunger is satiated)*
AUTONOMIC	• *Chest recession, breathing or heart rate increasing or decreasing, colour changes (responses which indicate inability to cope)*
MOTOR	• *Tensing or turning head away (eg. to reject food)*
NON-VERBAL	• *Eye widening or facial grimace (as reaction to strong-tasting food)*
VOCAL	• *Vocalizing (eg. to ask for more food)*
GESTURAL	• *Pushing away with the hand (eg. to reject food)*
VERBAL	• *Says "drink" (eg. to request same)*
BEHAVIOURAL	• *Screams (eg. to get attention or favourite food)*

Some of these behaviours will be responses to stimuli (non-intentional) and some will be deliberate. This will depend on the child's cognitive, physical and behavioural difficulties.

23

Not all behaviours are communication acts and it is important to determine whether a behaviour is actually functioning as a communication (as a response, or to convey information). Use of the last two columns in the checklist will help in this exercise. For example, by evaluating what precedes a behaviour, the clinician can identify whether specific actions result in specific responses from the child. An example of this would be the feeder placing the spoon far back on the tongue, producing an arching response from the child. The last column, which looks at the feeder's response, can help identify whether particular feeder reactions are maintaining inappropriate behaviours, and whether the feeder is reading the child's communication signals.

Therapy guidelines

1 ··· It is important to **determine the origin and function of the behavioural/communication act**. Observed acts may fall into a number of categories, as follows:

▼ **the child's intentional communication signals;**
▼ **the child's non-intentional communication signals;**
▼ **part of the feeder–child interaction pattern;**
▼ **multifactorial – a combination of categories.**

Observation and discussion are a great help, as is:

▼ **The use of checklists (see the 'Stress Behaviours Checklist' or the 'Communication Behaviours Checklist'). Winstock (1994) has devised a communication checklist for use at feeding time;**
▼ **Analysis of responses to multisensory stimuli (auditory, visual, tactile, olfactory and gustatory) can also give good indications of a child's communication pattern;**
▼ **Videotaping a feeding session for subsequent analysis is often useful as the feeder is able to relax and watch the session, rather than being actively involved, as during feeding time.**

2 ··· Where the child refuses to feed, do not force-feed. This is, of course, possible but never recommended as the child becomes passive and feeding becomes a negative experience. Once this happens, it can be extremely difficult to advance the child's feeding development. The golden rule is: be **persistent and consistent**.

3 ··· **Establish a routine.** This will help the child predict and understand the feeding process and the boundaries contained within.

▼ **have set times;**
▼ **use consistent feeders;**
▼ **confine feeding to one room or place;**
▼ **use the same equipment: for example, high chair, table.**

4 · · · **Establish a rhythm** to feeding. This will help the child predict and understand what happens during feeding time. This will include, for example, presenting a loaded spoon once every minute (depending on the child) or once the child has swallowed, and placing it in front of the child's mouth.

5 · · · Never prolong feeding: **set a time limit**, which should never be more than half an hour. This functions to help the child predict and understand the feeding process as well as the adult's intentions. A lengthier feeding time will serve to undermine the process, causing further negative feeling about feeding. Setting a time limit may also have a further positive benefit, as the child may become hungrier more quickly, increasing his desire for food for the next time. If nutrition and calorie intake are a problem, they can be supplemented through tube feedings where appropriate, or smaller, more frequent, meals can be implemented.

6 · · · Outside of mealtimes, **allow food play**. This will serve to take the pressure from feeding and create a more relaxed feeling about it.

▼ **Use a plastic bath or mat and place utensils and foods of sloppy and other child-appropriate textures in it.**
▼ **Allow the child to be as messy as possible. A child can put his hands to food from about age six months and is able to explore it by prodding and squeezing from age nine months.**
▼ **Have finger foods available for the child where appropriate.**
▼ **Encourage and demonstrate 'pretend' play with dolls, teddy bears and utensils. This behaviour develops from about 12 months, becoming more refined as the child matures.**
▼ **Make feeding more stimulating by having the child's favourite toy – teddy, dinosaur, doll – take part in the actual feeding.**

7 · · · Where the child is not distracted or hypersensitive, **make feeding a sociable activity** involving peers and other family members. While some physically disabled children have their own particular seats, every effort should be made to have them part of a group around the table, rather than fed separately or alone. If this is not possible, the child should still be involved in the interaction that occurs at mealtimes by sitting with others and having finger foods or sloppy foods present (for social, not nutritional reasons), whichever is appropriate.

8 · · · **Ensure there is no audience** (that is, peers and family members) for inappropriate behaviours. Advise all people to respond consistently; turn attention away from negative behaviours.

9 · · · **Focus on main meals** as the only source of eating by eliminating snacks or eating between meals. This is particularly relevant where children are fussy or junk food eaters.

25

10 ·· **Reinforce behaviours appropriately.** Do not respond to negative behaviours, but signal verbally that you have recognized them. Inappropriate responding, whether it is negative or positive, will only serve to reinforce behaviours because they gain attention. Reinforce and praise appropriate behaviours; this will serve to encourage the child, provide attention for appropriate skills and maximize positive behaviours. For example, "You closed your lips then, well done." Reinforce the entire feeding session, when appropriate, by doing a favourite activity with the child after the feeding is finished.

11 ·· Where there is a behavioural/control element to feeding, **use strategies adapted specifically to the situation**. These strategies will mean that feeding time does not become a battleground; they turn attention away from the negative behaviours and help the child understand that the adult is in control and will set boundaries. This approach will not be successful if the feeder becomes angry or upset, or is unable to maintain the strategy, as this will mean that the child has regained control.

▼ **Do not display emotion except when it comes to praising the child for eating and so on.**

▼ **When the behaviour is food refusal, have the feeder remove herself from the situation. Comment on the child's behaviour: for example, "You are telling me you are not ready to eat"; explain what you will do: "So I will finish the washing up." The feeder should leave for a couple of minutes and return, presenting the spoon again. If the reaction is the same, the feeder should act in the above manner again. When the 20–30 minutes for the mealtime is up, the food should be removed and feeding ended.**

▼ **When the child refuses to eat, remain with the feeding, remaining in position. For example, if the child closes their mouth when a spoon is produced, the feeder can hold the spoon an inch from the mouth and wait. It is important to advise the child that the feeder will wait. If this is prolonged, put down the spoon, move to another activity such as washing up, and then return.**

▼ **With a child who is beginning to feed himself but is reluctant to do so, encourage the 'one more spoon' approach. If the child will only take one spoon before expecting the feeder to feed him the rest, encourage and help him to take just one more spoon and then continue to feed him. This can be extended and graded as appropriate: for example, one extra spoon each week.**

12 ·· **Grade changes** if a child's system is hypersensitive and the behaviour is a coping reaction.

13 ·· **Use distracters,** such as toys and rattles. This strategy works well with some children by removing their attention from the feeding process, but negatively with others, who lose interest in eating.

14 ·· Where appropriate, **use choice making** to give the child some choice and control in the session. For example, ask "Do you want a drink or a chip?"

15 ·· Encourage the feeder to **develop a positive mind-set** before the session, eg. through mental imaging.

16 ·· **Help the child to regard the session, and feeding in general, positively** by telling constructive, confident and happy stories with food themes. Use storybooks; tell stories of good food occasions such as picnics and so on; use videos.

17 ·· **Consult a clinical psychologist** where appropriate.

Overview

Function and Effects

As the cheeks provide the lateral boundaries of the oral cavity and they work closely with the lips, any problems with the cheeks can affect the labial area, causing problems such as poor lip seal/closure; reduced ability to produce pressure or suction (particularly important in breast and bottle feeding); excessive liquid loss; and reduced ability to facilitate good bolus formation.

In young infants, the sucking pads (fat pads) will help provide cheek stability and therefore lip flexion and seal.

Causes and Contributory Factors

Problems in this area can arise as a result of orofacial hypotonia and weakness; and small or diminished fat pads in young infants.

Therapy guidelines

1. ··· **Correct positioning** will provide increased overall stability and control. The focus should be on flexion and symmetry. Neck elongation and chin tuck will help the lips to be more active in suction or food removal. See 'Positioning' guidelines (pages 82–83).

2. ··· **Stimulate improved cheek tone.** Movements should be firm, gentle and quick, but rhythmical. Use tapping, patting, stroking, vibration or quick stretches. Play games such as 'pat-a-cake' and 'peek-a-boo' on the cheeks. Encourage the child to use his hands to stimulate and increase awareness of this area. Use music to establish a rhythm (see Evans-Morris and Dunn-Klein, 1987). See 'Orofacial Hypotonia' guidelines (pages 79–81).

3. ··· **Provide added sensory input.** Expand and increase the range of foods and tastes available to the child (for example, different sauces). This will also serve to increase pleasure and interest.

   Explore distinct textures (different textured cloths and toys) and shapes (toys and objects) with hands, face and mouth.

4. ··· **Develop oro-motor skills** to develop lip and cheek control and strength.

a] **Blowing games.**

▼ Use candles, bubbles, whistles, pin wheels, a football game using light tissue paper for the ball, light stickers which can be used for reinforcement, paper snowballs or packing material to make a snowstorm and so on.

▼ Demonstrate using exaggerated lip movements.

▼ Initially have the object as near as is safely possible to the child's lips.

▼ Increase the distance as the child's strength develops.

b] **Straws.**

▼ Use straws if appropriate: usually the child is able to use straws by age three years (Arvedson and Christensen, 1993) but individuals vary and some children can use straws by 18 months.

▼ Use straws of differing thickness, length, shapes and angles to help with cheek tone and stability.

▼ As the child develops, increase the difficulty and therefore the effort required.

▼ Use squeeze bottle drinks initially – they are easier to suck from. Help the child in the beginning by squeezing the container slightly.

▼ Use liquids of differing consistencies – level 1 (thin), such as water, to level 2 (thick), such as milkshakes (see page 39).

▼ Use a range of tastes for enjoyment and reinforcement. Play guessing games by hiding the contents. Encourage the child to guess what the liquid is.

c] **Cold stimulation and sucking.**

▼ Sucking (not licking) cold/long foods such as lollipops/frozen juice sticks, refrigerated slices of fruit or liquorice sticks will aid closure.

▼ Make this more difficult by reducing the size of objects presented.

5 ··· **Provide external support.** Support to the cheeks and lips may help increase lip approximation around the teat or spoon. Place the thumb and index finger on the cheeks and facilitate lip pursing (Evans-Morris and Dunn-Klein, 1987; Wolf and Glass, 1992). Jaw support may also be needed with some infants. This may be easier with a small bottle which can be supported between the thumb and index finger, leaving the other fingers free to support the jaw (Wolf and Glass, 1992).

6 ··· With bottle-fed children, if sucking activity is observed but intake is minimal, **ensure a good latch** is achieved by checking that the lower lip is curled outwards, and that the lips approximate the fatter base of the teat. Facilitate directly if necessary or try a different teat.

7 ··· **Place food in cheek pockets** where appropriate, to encourage the child to use the cheeks to retrieve it.

Overview

Chewing is a complex process which involves the co-ordination of the lips, tongue, cheeks and jaw. Arvedson (1993a, page 147) describes chewing as 'a process used to break up solids with lateral, spreading and rolling movements of the tongue propelling food between the teeth, and rotary movements of the jaw'.

Normal Development

The guidelines below are based on Arvedson (1993a), Evans-Morris and Dunn-Klein (1987) and Winstock (1994). The child continues to suck food until around age nine months. Early chewing (biting) starts at six months and is an acquired skill, not a reflex action. Munching/vertical chewing (vertical tongue and jaw movements) is the first to develop. This is followed by a gradual development in diagonal chewing (across the midline of the oral cavity, using lateral tongue and jaw movements) and circular (rotary) chewing.

The child is able to chew relatively efficiently by 18 months–two years, when he has a sustained controlled bite with appropriate lip seal. Food spillage may continue until age three years.

Therapy guidelines

1 ··· **Reduce environmental overstimulation.** Too many stimuli can increase tension in the child and a lack of concentration on the feeding process.

2 ··· **Concentrate on the main problem area** which can constrain the development of chewing. Target limiting movements of any of the structures (jaw, lips, cheeks, tongue). See relevant sections. Additionally, an intolerance to lumps may be a contributory factor. (See 'Food Consistency' guidelines on page 39.)

3 ··· **Provide preparatory handling** which can reduce tone. This is particularly relevant as chewing can contribute to patterns of increased tension, because it is a more complex oro-motor pattern. Use gentle rocking. Play calm music. Massage the muscles of mastication (above and below the zygomatic arch) before feeding as this will prepare the child for chewing. Use fingers or a vibrator. Try this technique if the child has a tonic bite reflex, as this can

30

sometimes affect appropriate chewing. Before the introduction of food, manipulate the jaw forwards, backwards and laterally. Once the food is in the mouth, the jaw can be directly manipulated laterally to encourage and support chewing. Consult the child's paediatric occupational therapist or physiotherapist.

4 ··· **Provide correct positioning,** which should help reduce limiting patterns and hypertonicity and contribute to stability so that the child's jaw can be steady and ready to accept food. Emphasize flexion and chin tuck; ensure symmetrical alignment. (See 'Positioning' guidelines, pages 82–83.)

5 ··· **Provide mouthing experience and practice.** Use the child's own hands to facilitate placement in the mouth. Use rubber toys with appendages for biting to help develop control.

6 ··· **Facilitate, demonstrate and practise the correct pattern.**

▼ **Exaggerate using an open mouth posture.**
▼ **Use a mirror to provide visual feedback.**
▼ **Demonstrate yawning, laughing, blowing, pouting, making faces and so on (Evans-Morris and Dunn-Klein, 1987).**
▼ **During feeding, show the child the correct chewing movements and pattern. Encourage the child to imitate.**

7 ··· Evans-Morris and Dunn-Klein (1987) recommend the **stimulation of the lateral borders of the tongue**. This should provide a stimulus for more advanced chewing patterning. Do this directly by using a finger, wet cotton swab, toothbrush or foods such as breadsticks. Start feeding by positioning the spoon centrally and then placing it to the side of the mouth between the gum ridges.

8 ··· **Stimulate biting skills.**

▼ **Start with foods that are easy to bite and chew and increase the firmness as the child develops improved patterning. Foods which dissolve in the mouth, such as prawn crackers or sponge fingers, are ideal. Alexander (1987) recommends foods such as cheese and crackers.**
▼ **Use foods that allow for a continuous bite (long and thin) such as liquorice sticks, bread sticks, dried fruit strips, strips of beef, chips and strips of semi-cooked carrot and, if appropriate (no swallowing dysfunction), try sugarless gum (Evans-Morris and Dunn-Klein, 1987; Winstock, 1994).**
▼ **For a hypertonic child use softer foods. For a hypotonic child, use firmer foods (Winstock, 1994).**

▼ If a tonic bite reflex is present and the likelihood is that the food will be bitten off, place moistened gauze-wrapped food in the cheek pocket or on the gum/dental ridges.

▼ Start feeding by positioning the spoon centrally and then placing it to the side of the mouth between the gum ridges.

9 ⋯ **Provide the stimulus for chewing.**
Use appropriately sized utensils and boluses: too large may cause gagging or restrict tongue movement; too small may not provide enough sensory information and therefore stimulus for change. A narrow spoon will introduce less food and more control, leading to more appropriate patterning (Evans-Morris and Dunn-Klein, 1987; Winstock, 1994). Use foods that require chewing. Liquid, mashed or puréed consistencies will not encourage chewing. Start by thickening the consistency and continue from there. (See 'Food Consistency' guidelines, page 41.)

10 ⋅⋅ **Use dry and sweet foods** where possible and appropriate, as this will develop patterning and control. These foods will require more effort and increase the production of saliva, which will promote chewing.

11 ⋅⋅ **Eliminate practices which do not promote appropriate patterning and produce limiting patterns.** Presenting food at a suitable temperature will encourage a less reactive and more controlled response (Evans-Morris and Dunn-Klein, 1987). Extremes of temperature will result in extreme reactions. Do not scrape the spoon against the teeth or gum ridge as this tends to encourage a sucking rather than chewing pattern, and will contribute to increased tone and extension.

12 ⋅⋅ Gradually **increase the range of flavours** in terms of strength, taste and consistency. This will provide more sensory input and more mature eating skills.

13 ⋅⋅ **Provide opportunities for food play** and exploration which will encourage a more relaxed attitude to feeding and food.

▼ With younger children, messy food on a slip mat or plastic child's bath can be fun.

▼ Finger food should be left around the house and be available for the child to taste and explore spontaneously.

▼ Take turns with hiding food in the adult's and child's mouth and transferring from side to side.

▼ Focus on pretend play with dolls and teddy bears and toy utensils. The child can play at feeding others, including the feeder.

Overview

Causes and Contributory Factors

A cleft lip results from failure of fusion of the upper lip in the fifth week of embryonic development, and a cleft palate from failure of fusion of the palatal shelves in the midline in the seventh to eighth week. These conditions can occur individually or together, unilaterally or bilaterally, and vary in the degree of severity.

Function

The hard palate works with the tongue to compress the teat or nipple to maintain its position. The soft palate helps create the posterior seal. When elevated, the soft palate seals the nasal cavity, allowing food to pass into the oesophagus and preventing nasal reflux.

Implications

The degree of feeding difficulty may depend on the child's specific anatomical, airway and neurological factors (Arvedson, 1993a). Swallowing function and tongue and jaw movements are generally adequate in these children, but they may need a focus on their feeding because they may present with difficulties in producing suction, slow weight gain and nasal reflux.

Therapy guidelines

1 ··· **Surgical intervention** at six weeks to four months for closure of the lip and at 12 to 18 months generally for closure of the palate.

2 ··· **Correct positioning** – with the focus on good support. An upright or half-sitting position will allow the liquid to move into the pharynx and away from the nasal cavity.

3 ··· **A suitable teat** and/or specialized bottle will ensure that the liquid does not flow upwards into the nasal cavity. Arvedson (1993a) recommends a wide-based, flat teat that occludes the cleft by pressing against it, although this may not be as effective with larger clefts, or a soft teat with modifications, such as an enlarged or cross-cut hole. A specialized bottle such as the Haberman feeder is also suitable. See Winstock (1994) for stockists.

33

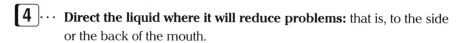

4 ··· **Direct the liquid where it will reduce problems:** that is, to the side or the back of the mouth.

5 ··· **Prevent tiredness and energy expenditure.** Start with small and more frequent feedings, rather than larger meals. Establish a rhythm, fast enough to prevent fatigue and slow enough to give more control and prevent gagging and choking.

6 ··· Prevent or **reduce nasal reflux**. A small amount of reflux may not interfere significantly with feeding. See 'Nasal Reflux' guidelines (page 109).

7 ··· **Monitor weight gain,** as these children are often slow to put on weight. Supplements or increased fat diet may be necessary. See 'Increasing Nutritional Intake' guidelines (pages 72–73). Refer to a paediatric dietician.

8 ··· **Provide frequent winding** (Arvedson, 1993a).

9 ··· **Consider a palatal prosthesis** to close the cleft temporarily. This can be made by a specialist clinic or experienced paediatric dental surgeon. Views differ about the use of prostheses, but Arvedson (1993a) states that a palatal prosthesis may be considered for a child with a wide unilateral or bilateral cleft of the lip and palate.

10 ·· If the mother is **breast-feeding**, this has the best prognosis with a narrow posterior palatal cleft, or a submucous cleft of the soft palate (Arvedson, 1993a). The prognosis is poorest with a large palatal cleft.

Overview

Normal Development: Oro-motor Skills

The transition to cup drinking normally happens around the time that the child is first introduced to puréed foods, at four to six months of age. A sucking or suckling pattern usually continues until about 18 months, when an up–down tongue pattern emerges. Stability is first achieved by placing the tongue underneath the cup. At 18 months, biting the cup is the stability strategy. External control is usually achieved by age two years, in line with improved jaw stability.

Normal Development: Self-feeding Skills

Work on cup drinking is not appropriate if the child has not reached the developmental age of about four to six months, when he can support cup drinking with the aid of an adult who holds the cup. From six to nine months, the child will put his hands to a cup and may hold it, but spillage may continue to happen up to age 18 months. One-handed drinking normally occurs by age two years (Winstock, 1994).

Therapy guidelines

1 ⋯ **Ensure positioning** that provides the support and stability necessary for cup drinking. See 'Positioning' guidelines (pages 82–83).

2 ⋯ **Ensure jaw stability.** It is important for the child's jaw to be steady in preparation for the cup. Demonstrate a quiet, steady mouth (Evans-Morris and Dunn-Klein, 1987).

Stand behind the child and support his jaw with the palm of one hand. Tip the cup with the other hand. If necessary, support the lower lip with the index finger of the hand supporting the jaw.

Encourage internal stability, if appropriate, by having the child hold on to the cup by biting the rim with his teeth. Do not use this strategy with a child with a tonic bite reflex.

Maintain constant contact between the cup and the lower lip. Do not keep removing it during feeding, even when the child stops drinking (Evans-Morris and Dunn-Klein, 1987). A cup with a weighted base may provide stability (Winstock, 1994).

Be consistent and establish a rhythm. (See recommendations below.)

35

Let the child see the bolus before feeding.

Work on lip closure (see 'Lip Seal' guidelines, pages 61–63).

See also 'Jaw Stability' guidelines (pages 57–58).

3 ··· Winstock (1994) recommends trying **an empty cup** before introducing it into a real feeding situation. This is an enjoyable and non-threatening way to introduce cups. Do functional and 'pretend' play. Use dolls, utensils, the adult and the child. Demonstrate how a cup is used by placing it to the doll's lips, teddy bear, adult and so on.

4 ··· When introducing drinking from cups, **start with familiar and especially well-liked flavours**.

5 ··· **Expand the range and strength of tastes** available to the child while he is still using a bottle: for example, juices such as apple, carrot, tomato and apricot.

6 ··· **Try out different cups.** Warner (1981) recommends using a small cup from a tea set, or a medicine cup, whose size will not put the child off. Additionally, the amount of liquid presented to the child in such cups is reduced, which may help with control of the contents. A cup with a weighted base may provide stability (Winstock, 1994). A medicine cup, a beaker squeezed to form a spout or a Doidy cup may help with control of the liquid.

Training cups can be used to grade the development of cup drinking: for example, from a spout to a cup with a slit or hole, to an open-topped cup. A child with a tonic bite reflex will have this pattern exacerbated by spouted cups.

A wide-lipped cup helps the child to see the drink. Consult the child's paediatric occupational therapist about the range of cups available.

7 ··· Have the **cup at least half-full**, but do not overfill. The natural tendency is to fill the cup, but this often results in spillage. A half-full cup will help with control.

8 ··· **Eliminate feeder practices which may contribute to limiting patterns.** Do not press down on the lower lip, but on the anterior tongue. Direct the liquid to the upper corner of the mouth, gently touching the lower lip. Do not pour the fluid into the child's mouth.

9 ··· **Establish a rhythm** which helps the child predict and control the feeding process, the utensil and its contents. Preparatory handling through gentle rocking, particularly where a child is hypersensitive, can relax and steady the child. Use calming music. Provide verbal cues such as 'drink' and 'stop'.

10 ·· **Thicken the consistency** of the drink, particularly in the initial stages, to help develop control. Use thick liquids (level 2) such as pineapple juice. Try puréed but watered down food. Purée home-blended fruit or vegetables. Try milkshakes.

Gradually thin the drink by watering down, using level 1 liquids (for example water, apple juice) as appropriate and necessary.

11 ·· **Move at the child's pace.** Monitor and respond to the child's communication signals through whichever mode they are made. This will help the child trust the feeder and enable the process to develop.

37

Overview

Normal Development

Transition from liquids to solids usually follows the developmental pattern outlined below, based on Warner (1981). The development of motor skills, including head control and general stability, leads the way for the development of the more advanced and fine motor and oro-motor skills.

From birth to three months: liquids only

From three to six months: introduction of puréed (smooth, semi-solid) foods, particularly cereals.

From six to nine months: mashed foods are added; finger foods are used under guidance.

From 12 months: coarsely chopped, firmer textured foods, including some meats; a greater range of tastes is used.

From 18 months: most meats and raw vegetables.

Causes and Contributory Factors

It is important to rely on the child's developmental rather than chronological age as a guideline. Transition difficulties can be caused or contributed to by a number of factors, such as behaviour, orofacial tone problems, orofacial hypersensitivity, and the presence of a gag reflex.

A recent study by Reilly *et al* (1995) demonstrated that texture had an important influence on oro-motor skills, and the use of thicker and more adult-like texture affected the food refusal rate in children studied.

There has been and there remains controversy over the labels usually ascribed to food consistencies. In light of this, it may be more beneficial to talk of food consistencies in steps rather than using adjectives which are open to subjective interpretation (see 'Food Consistency Levels', below). Additionally, this approach recognizes a greater variety and makes development in this area easier to identify and, perhaps, easier to facilitate. It is intended to be developmental in nature but it must be noted, for example, that some children will move on to finger foods and semi-solids concurrently. Also finger foods can comprise different food consistencies. Using this approach may also help to generalize, but, when talking about an individual child, the most important consideration is between the clinician and team members to maintain consistency.

Use the checklist to evaluate what food consistency level the child has reached. Ask the parent to prepare in advance, using the 'Food Diary' on page 71, a list of exactly what the child has eaten over three days. Write the listed foods in the appropriate boxes. This will give the clinician an idea of what level the child's main intake falls under.

FOOD CONSISTENCY LEVELS

FOOD LEVEL	FOOD TYPE
Level 1	*Light liquids, eg. thin untextured soup, untextured thin juices (apple and grape), water*
Level 2	*Heavy liquids, eg. condensed untextured soup, yogurt, milkshake, custard, soft icecream, thicker juices (tomato and pineapple)*
Level 3	*Thin purées (blends) of any type or combination of foods, whether commercial or home-blended*
Level 4	*Thick purées, less blended than above, or thickened by adding, for example, baby cereal, icecream or mashed banana to yogurt or fromage frais.*
Level 5	*Mashed foods, eg. vegetables, banana, avocado, scrambled egg, soft boiled egg*
Level 6	*Semi–solids, eg. apple sauce, semolina, grated apple to cereal, soft flaked fish, blended meat and mashed vegetables added to mashed potatoes*
Level 7	*Finger foods, eg. semi-cooked strips of carrot, soft cheese squares, toast 'soldiers' (strips of toast), melt-in-the-mouth foods such as prawn crackers*
Level 8	*Solids, eg. most ordinary family meals such as spaghetti*
Level 9	*Chewables, eg. raisins, chicken, canned beans, hard cheese*
Level 10	*Tougher chewables, eg. meats, raw vegetables, hard sweets*
Level 11	*Mixed textures, eg. vegetable soups, adult cereals with milk, minced meat in sauce*

39

▼

FOOD CONSISTENCY LEVEL CHECKLIST

NAME	DATE

LEVEL	FOODS TAKEN
Level 1 (thin liquids)	
Level 2 (thick liquids)	
Level 3 (thin purées)	
Level 4 (thick purées)	
Level 5 (mashed foods)	
Level 6 (semi-solids)	
Level 7 (finger foods)	
Level 8 (solids)	
Level 9 (chewables)	
Level 10 (tough chewables)	
Level 11 (mixed textures)	

MAIN CONSISTENCY LEVEL

Therapy guidelines

1 · · · Always **taste the food** yourself before introducing it to the child. Check for oversaltiness, sweetness, sourness and so on.

2 · · · Until the child has the appropriate skills, **do not use foods of mixed consistencies**, such as minestrone soup (a combination of liquid and solids).

3 · · · **Use home-cooked foods** which are less sweet than commercial brands. This will make the progression to more solid food easier. Use a blender to achieve this.

4 · · · When upgrading the consistency, **thicken foods** by using thicker liquids; adding baby cereal, cornflour and water mixture, or reducing the liquid content through cooking and/or adding less liquid; or making foods which are less blended than previously.

5 · · · Have **finger foods** if appropriate, readily available or casually placed around the house, so that the child can explore and taste them at his own pace. Do not direct the child to the finger foods, or pressurize him to eat them.

6 · · · To ease the presentation of new foods, **introduce new tastes in small amounts** initially. This applies at all levels of food transition.

▼ **Dip a dummy/pacifier or finger into liquids and purées and let the child explore the taste.**
▼ **Dilute new or strong tastes, such as juices, with water at first.**
▼ **Add a spoonful of the new flavour to the child's milk or yogurt.**
▼ **When the child becomes used to the new tastes, thicken the consistency by reducing the water content or increasing the concentration of the new flavour.**
▼ **Cut solid foods into small lumps, gradually increasing the size of lump.**
▼ **Always monitor the child's reaction.**

7 · · · **Make feeding sociable** rather than an isolated activity with attention focused only on the child. Have the child sit with peers at drinks time, or with the family at mealtime. Even if the intention is not for the child to eat, place a plate of food in front of him just as with the rest of the family.

Do not focus on the child's refusal or avoidance of food. Carry on normal mealtime activities or conversations. If the child tries the food, praise him in one short sentence, such as "Well done, you licked the chip." Do not overpraise the child. One comment is sufficient.

41

Overview

Normal Development

The gag reflex (a protective laryngeal cough) occurs in response to stimulation in the oral area and is important for safe feeding. It is particularly sensitive in the newborn and gradually becomes less sensitive from nine to 12 months (Winstock, 1994) as the place where the gag is elicited in the oral cavity moves progressively back. The gag reflex is still evident in adulthood, but individuals vary in their sensitivity, and where it can be elicited varies from person to person.

Causes and Contributory Factors

Excessive gagging, coughing or choking can indicate a number of problems. Most significant is a swallowing dysfunction. Problems with swallowing can result in food remaining in the oropharyngeal area causing choking. Sensation problems can also contribute. Children who are hypotonic or have a history of naso- or orogastric tube feeding, for example, may be desensitized in the oropharyngeal area, with reduced control over the bolus resulting. Hypersensitivity in this area can result in gagging reactions to food, again reducing control over the bolus.

A gag reflex may be especially prevalent in children with chewing problems (Winstock, 1994). Gagging and choking can occur as the child makes food transitions, particularly to more solid textures: new textures are new tactile experiences. As tolerance develops, the incidence of gagging and choking decreases (Alexander, 1987).

Classification

Winstock (1994) classifies gagging behaviour into four main areas. Each classification has implications for the way food is handled in the oral cavity.

1 ··· Hypersensitive – too easily and readily stimulated (for example, elicited at the tongue tip or lips).

2 ··· Hyposensitive – not stimulated as quickly as normal when food is in the oral cavity.

3 ··· Absent – no gag reflex present. Potential for aspiration is increased.

4 ··· Delayed/suppressed – the child needs to gag but abnormal muscle tone inhibits this function. The need to gag can be seen in these children in blinking or watering eyes and similar responses.

Gagging can be rated for severity into mild, moderate, severe or profound. The ratings below are guidelines and help in recording progress resulting from therapy input and medical management, and the severity of gagging or choking. These ratings are useful as long as a clinician applies them consistently to an individual child. Where teams are concerned, they need to agree on what constitutes each level. Suggested ratings are based on a number of factors: (1) frequency of occurrence; (2) disruption to the feeding process and child recovery; (3) effects on nutritional intake; and (4) what elicits the gag, and where it is elicited. It is important to note that other factors may be affecting the feeding process and having an impact on these areas.

Grading

GRADE	CHARACTERISTICS
0 Normal	*No problems with gagging or choking or desensitization observed*
1 Mild	*Infrequent: gagging occurs occasionally or does not occur sometimes when necessary* • *Child recovers rapidly* • *Feeding not lengthy* • *Intake and weight gain not significantly affected* • *Presence or absence of gagging not affected by differing food consistencies* • *Gag elicited as normal in posterior portion of tongue (except for infants)*
2 Moderate	*Gagging occurs or is not observed when necessary a few times during feeding* • *Recovery not immediate but not excessively prolonged* • *Feeding relatively lengthy relative to intake* • *Intake reduced and weight gain affected but this is not threatening* • *Gag elicited or reduced by particular food consistencies* • *Gag elicited in middle-anterior portion of the tongue/absent or reduced on posterior portion of tongue*

3 Severe	*Occurs or absent every session a number of times* • *Recovery prolonged and slow* • *Feeding excessively lengthy and tiring for feeder and child.* • *Nutritional intake and weight gain significantly affected and a cause for continuing concern and monitoring* • *Gag stimulated/absent on all food consistencies* • *Gag elicited at anterior portion of mouth (lips, anterior tongue)/reduced or absent in tonsillar area*
4 Profound	*Gagging is frequent or continual or absent constantly* • *Recovery excessively prolonged* • *Feeding significantly disrupted by occurrence or absence of gagging* • *Nutritional intake and weight gain significantly compromised* • *Gag stimulated or absent on all food consistencies* • *Gag elicited at face and anterior portion of mouth (lips) or absent in oropharyngeal area* • *Oral feeding contraindicated*

Use the checklist to help evaluate why gagging or choking occurs and to analyse the surrounding issues.

GAGGING AND CHOKING CHECKLIST

NAME	DATE

Part 1: *Causal Factors*

PROBLEM AREA	PRESENT	ABSENT
SENSATION		
Oropharyngeal hyposensitivity		
Oropharyngeal hypersensitivity		
ORO–MOTOR		
Poor co-ordination of the suck – swallow – breathe pattern		
Delayed swallow reflex		
Exaggerated gag reflex		
MEDICAL		
Respiratory problems		
Reduced endurance		
MOTOR		
Orofacial hypotonia		
Orofacial hypertonia		
ASSOCIATED CONDITIONS		
Aspiration		
Reflux		
BEHAVIOURAL		
Used as attention-seeking strategy		
Dependent on feeder response		

Part 2: *Triggers*

QUESTION	ANSWER
Do the specific utensils used trigger episodes?	
Does gagging/choking occur or increase in severity with a specific feeder?	
What precedes episodes of gagging or choking?	

45

Part 3: *Severity*

QUESTION	ANSWER
How quickly does the child recover from episodes?	
To what extent is feeding disrupted by presence or absence of gagging and choking? How long does it take to feed the child an ounce/millilitre?	
Is nutritional intake compromised? Is intake reduced during sessions? How is weight gain?	
What food consistencies affect the occurrence or absence of gagging or choking? Solids, purées, liquids (see gradings on page 39).	
Where is gag elicited? Lips, anterior, middle, posterior portion of tongue or oropharynx?	
Is gagging or choking absent when necessary or frequent (indicating aspiration)? Note the number of episodes per spoon/amount of food given.	
Rate severity: Grade 0, 1, 2, 3, or 4	

Part 4: *Summary*

QUESTION	ANSWER
Is gagging primarily hypersensitive, hyposensitive, absent, suppressed or behavioural in origin?	

Therapy guidelines

1 ··· **Check swallowing function** through observation and touch. Place your hands around the area of the hyoid bone. It should move up and down in time with a swallow. This technique usually works best with children whose swallows are fairly intact. However, even if movement is not felt, the co-ordination and timing of the swallow or swallows will provide valuable information.

Place your hands under the chin where the floor of the mouth and the root of the tongue meet. As the tongue is intimately involved in the swallowing process, it should be felt to rise and fall in time with a swallow. Lack of movement in this area will help in diagnosis.

Is saliva control reduced or can the child manage its oral secretions?

See guidelines on pages 119–121.

2 ··· **Refer for videofluoroscopy** where appropriate to determine:
(1) the extent of the problem (gagging can be particularly noticeable when using this technique, especially where the tongue humps);
(2) contributing oro-motor structures and functions;
(3) associated conditions such as reflux and/or aspiration.

3 ··· **Monitor the child's state** when doing feeding and prefeeding work. This will help you to anticipate problems.

▼ **Observe respiration at rest and during feeding. Watch for irregular patterns and shallow breathing.**
▼ **Observe motor behaviours and changes, including arching or sudden hypotonia.**
▼ **Observe for sudden drowsiness or alerting.**
▼ **Learn the child's communication signals.**
▼ **See the 'Stress Behaviours' checklist (page 20).**

4 ··· **Create a warm and relaxing prefeeding and feeding environment by:**

▼ **playing calming and slow music;**
▼ **telling stories;**
▼ **positive imaging of successful and happy feeding situations, such as picnics;**
▼ **rocking (Evans-Morris and Dunn-Klein, 1987);**
▼ **preventing and reducing negative experiences;**
▼ **reacting quickly but calmly when gagging occurs: this will help the child to construct the feeder positively, and will prevent frustration, anxiety and behavioural problems developing.**

5 ··· **Provide correct positioning** with the emphasis on chin tuck and general flexion. Gagging can be difficult when the chin is tucked.

47

▼

6 ··· **Develop internal control and strength.** Position the child appropriately, with emphasis on chin tuck. Develop more appropriate patterns of lip, tongue, cheek and jaw movement and function where these are poor. Reduce the negative, limiting patterns.

▼ **Develop breathing and phonatory control through blowing, singing and extended vocalizations (Arvedson, 1993b).**
▼ **Impose a sucking rhythm, as outlined in (8) below.**

7 ··· **Reduce the gag reflex.** Outside of feeding, use a finger, wet cotton swab, spatula/tongue depressor and so on. Use firm but gentle movements. Walk with the finger or a spatula (take small steps) from anterior to posterior of the tongue along the midline, stopping just before gag or hump is triggered. If the gag is elicited in the anterior portion of the tongue, begin in the gum ridge, labial or cheek area. Do this about five times, then stop. Repeat the activity several times a day. Move further back as the child's sensitivity decreases.

During feeding, gradually move the teat or spoon further back in the child's mouth as he becomes desensitized.

8 ··· **Establish a sucking rhythm.** Preparatory handling should include rocking and be accompanied by music.

With bottle feeding, observe the child's suck – swallow – breathe pattern and remove the teat before the gag occurs. Impose an external rhythm based on the child's abilities. For example, if the child gags after three sucks, break the suction at two sucks. The dictated rhythm will help with control. Gradually let the child take more control.

9 ··· **Eliminate practices or utensils that contribute to the pattern.** Use a short, small teat or spoon (Winstock, 1994; Wolf and Glass, 1992). Place the bolus or utensil appropriately – not too far back. Reduce the size of the bolus. A large bolus may limit tongue movement. Try cup drinking instead of bottle feeding where appropriate. Reduce the liquid content of the food by thickening it.

10 ·· With some children, when food is stuck, Warner (1981) recommends a gentle, firm, quick push in and up under the ribs, which will **encourage an expiratory breath** and help dislodge food. If trying this, make sure that it does not contribute to limiting patterns or respiratory compromise.

11 ·· **Use distractions** such as stories, singing toys or observations, in general directing the child's attention to something else in the environment.

12 ·· **Provide opportunities for food play** which will encourage the child to relax about food and feeding, and give greater feelings of control. With younger children, sloppy food on a plastic mat or plastic bath can be fun. Finger food should be left available for the child to explore when ready. Feeder and child take turns at hiding food or imaginary items in each other's mouths. 'Pretend' play with dolls and teddy bears. Use 'pretend' utensils and food if available.

13 ·· **Increase the child's tolerance and awareness of different tastes.** Introduce new tastes, one at a time. If the child is extremely sensitive, add one spoon to a food which he currently eats, such as yogurt, increasing this as the child grows accustomed to the new taste. Experiment along the opposite poles of taste such as sour and sweet.

14 ·· **Evaluate the feeder's reactions to the episodes of gagging** to determine if there is a behavioural element, whether overlying dysfunctional patterns or the primary etiology. Is the feeder obviously anxious, angry or frustrated? Is the child's gagging attracting attention? If so, the feeder will need to remain calm and remove attention from the gagging. This can be done by reducing emotions and reactions, remaining silent, leaving the room until the coughing is finished (ensure that there is no swallowing dysfunction present if this is the preferred method) or explaining to the child that the feeder will wait until the gagging is complete.

49

THE JAW

Introduction

When looking at the structure and function of the jaw, it is always necessary to consider normal development. Children initially need some support in feeding as their muscle bulk and tone will not be sufficiently developed for internal control to suffice. The following checklist will help the clinician in judging jaw function and also in determining which area is the primary problem. Characteristics noted are usually or sometimes associated with the particular dysfunction. For an individual child to have a particular problem, that child does not necessarily need to present with all the characteristics outlined in the checklist.

JAW FUNCTION CHECKLIST

NAME		DATE	

Part 1: *Area of Difficulty*

AREA	PRESENT	ABSENT
JAW CLENCHING • Jaw instability • General hypertonia • Orofacial hypertonia • Extension patterns • Jaw remains stuck in closed position		
TONIC BITE REFLEX • Occurs in flexed (eg. chin tuck) position • Orofacial hypersensitivity • Hypertonia • Noticeably stronger with hard stimuli, eg. metal spoons		
JAW INSTABILITY • General hypotonia • Orofacial hypotonia • Orofacial paresis (weakness) • Reduced cheek (sucking) pads in infants • Extension patterns • Abnormal tongue movements • Reduced jaw elevation (sucking, munching and chewing patterns affected) • Reduced lip seal		
JAW THRUST • Sudden, forceful movement • Orofacial hypersensitivity • Neck hyperextension • Oral pain (eg. dental pain, gum infection) • Dislocation of temperomandibular joint (TMJ)		

AREA	PRESENT	ABSENT
BEHAVIOURAL • Consistent pattern • Particular antecedents provoke the response • No associated tension • History of early aversive feeding experiences • Feeder–child interactions dysfunctional		
STRUCTURE **(note structural problems)** • Micrognathia etc • Syndrome with associated structural maldevelopment of jaw		

Part 2: *Summary Observations*

QUESTION	ANSWER
Is jaw function affecting the feeding process? If so, how significantly does it do so?	
What characterizes jaw function in feeding (clenching, tonic bite reflex etc)?	
Are structural problems evident? If so, how does this affect feeding?	

Jaw clenching/tonic bite reflex overview

Normal Development

Infants have a normal phasic bite reflex which is gradually replaced by a volitional primary phasic bite and release (small, rhythmical movements) pattern from age three to six months. This control is achieved on soft foods at 12 months and on hard foods by 18 months, although the child may open his mouth wider than necessary to age 24 months and continue to have associated arm and leg movements and head extension to about age 21 months. By 24 months there is a controlled sustained bite (Evans-Morris and Dunn-Klein, 1987; Winstock, 1994).

Causes and Contributory Factors

It is important to identify whether the pattern is one of lack of spontaneous opening of the mouth (usually seen in premature babies) or whether there is tension involved which would indicate jaw clenching or a tonic bite reflex. Jaw clenching is described by Alexander (1987) as 'abnormal jaw closure which occurs as compensation for excessive jaw instability'. It is usually elicited by tactile stimulation to the biting surfaces (the gums and teeth). Jaw clenching can be (1) primarily dysfunctional, as in conditions of hypertonia; (2) compensatory, as in conditions of jaw instability, where it is used as a strategy to help oro-motor control; or (3) behavioural. It may function to control, for example to indicate that the child is not ready for the next mouthful of food, or that he has finished eating.

Winstock notes the characteristics of a tonic bite reflex (TBR): there is increased muscle tone associated with a flexed pattern; it usually starts suddenly and becomes stronger; the hands may be clenched in this pattern; and it may occur as a result of hypersensitivity or in response to food entering the oral cavity.

Therapy guidelines

1 ··· **Determine whether the pattern is an abnormal response or behavioural** in nature. This can be difficult to evaluate but there are a few guidelines which can help. The degree of tension is usually greater when it is an abnormal pattern. Evaluate the antecedents to assess the pattern's nature. With a tonic bite reflex, for example, hard utensils can contribute to or exacerbate the response.

Evaluate the function of the pattern. Mouth clenching as a behavioural act can function in two ways: as a non-intentional response (for example, to indicate dislike of food, or to indicate sufficient intake) or as an intentional communication (for example, to refuse food or to get parental reaction).

Evaluate the feeder response. Does it serve to encourage or contribute to the pattern?

53

2 ··· **Use preparatory handling,** of the whole body or solely the facial and oral areas, to reduce tone and hypersensitivity and to help the child with internal organization and control. This should be carried out before the feeding session and may include activities such as rocking, holding, swaddling, where appropriate, and use of relaxing music. See guidelines on pages 92–94.

3 ··· Position the child to **provide stability and support for movement of the jaw.** If the child presents with a tonic bite reflex which is part of the flexed pattern, place him in a slightly extended position. Winstock (1994) recommends breaking the symmetry by turning the head to one side when the clenching or bite occurs.

4 ··· **Reduce environmental stimuli** that may be overloading the child's system. This reduction in stimuli should also help the child to concentrate on feeding, to gain more feedback from the techniques used, and to develop more internal stability and control. Create a relaxing environment for the child; remove excess auditory stimuli, for example by turning off the television; reduce excessive visual stimuli such as bright sunlight; reduce combined stimuli such as the presence of extra people.

5 ··· **Normalize sensation** by facilitating and practising appropriate movements. Alexander (1987) reports that early, consistent presentation of slow, deep-pressure orotactile input can stimulate more normal responses to touch and reduce the potential for clenching and tonic biting. This pressure should be directed towards the gums, teeth, tongue and hard palate. Introduce graded pressure along the teeth or gum ridge using fingers, a spoon, a small toothbrush and so on, while maintaining the jaw in a slightly open position with the thumb putting gentle but firm downward pressure on the chin. Wolf and Glass (1992) recommend the following practice: firmly stroke the outer portion of the gum ridges, starting in the middle and stroking back along the gum, two or three times each side; pause between quadrants for a swallow to occur.

▼ **Provide tapping using small range finger movements to the mouth.**
▼ **Demonstrate and practise a steady jaw and quiet tongue ready to receive food.**
▼ **To encourage lip posturing, place fingers on the child's cheeks and draw them forward. Also, stroke the finger downwards from nose to top lip.**
▼ **Gradually increase the variety of tastes and strengths of food.**
▼ **Play games such as patting and peek-a-boo, that involve tapping and patting the TMJ and jaw muscle.**

6 ··· **Improve jaw stability** (see 'Jaw Stability' guidelines on pages 57–58).

7 ··· **Reduce practices which may contribute to the child's pattern.**
Placing the spoon centrally may contribute to the tonic bite reflex.
Present the food instead slightly to one side of the mouth (Winstock,
1994). Stimulate the lips rather than the teeth or jaw by placing the
food/spoon/cup on the lower lip, not on the teeth (Evans-Morris and
Dunn-Klein, 1987). Use utensils that do not cause the child discomfort
or exacerbate the tension of the pattern if present. Hard and brittle
spoons and spouts can contribute to the problem, so utensils used
should be less stimulating, but strong enough to cope with a tonic bite
reflex if present. Evans-Morris and Dunn-Klein (1987), and Winstock
(1994) recommend the use of a coated, plastic spoon which will not
harm the teeth or cause discomfort. Alexander (1987) recommends
the use of a tongue depressor to present food.

Finger feeding when appropriate may help in the child's control of
and coping with the feeding process, and reduce reaction to hard
materials.

8 ··· Where appropriate, **assist with mouth opening and bite release**.
Never force the mouth open. Never respond negatively to the pattern,
as children are sensitive to others' reactions and this may increase
frustration and anxiety and aggravate the problem. Explore the child's
ability to release or open without any assistance.

During the meal, wipe the child's face, from the TMJ to the lips.

Place the thumb on the bony part of the chin or the TMJ, and provide
gentle but firm downward pressure. Winstock (1994) recommends
pushing the chin up slightly with a finger to initiate release. Tap the
lips, teeth or the side of jaw. Continue while the mouth is open *(ibid)*.
Gently move the jaw from side to side in small excursions *(ibid)*.

Develop control over biting in the child who does not present with
TBR by encouraging him to hold a food such as a cracker or soft
biscuit (food with some give) between his teeth while you break off
the outside portion. Explain to the child what he needs to do and why
(ibid). Additionally, the feeder puts one end of a cloth in her mouth
and demonstrates a dog shaking the cloth. Then play a game of two
dogs trying to retain the cloth (Evans-Morris and Dunn-Klein, 1987).

Wait for the tension to pass.

9 ··· Focus on the **development of more advanced eating patterns**, such
as chewing, if appropriate. This will take the focus off a tense, biting
reaction and develop more control.

See 'Chewing' guidelines on pages 30–32.

10 ·· **Use rhythm, consistency and routine** to help the child predict and
control movements.

55

11 ·· **Make prefeeding time fun and relaxed.** Aim to diminish the tension. Provide an environment of mutual exploration of the feeder's and child's mouth. Activities could include counting teeth, comparing teeth, hiding food, searching for imaginary toys (Arvedson, 1993b).

Use utensils outside feeding time in 'pretend' play activities with dolls and teddy bears. The feeder can demonstrate, or the child can play at feeding others, including the feeder.

Use relaxing and favourite music before and during the session.

Tell stories that the child enjoys (Evans-Morris and Dunn-Klein, 1987). Stories about good food times such as picnics will help the child view feeding more positively.

Use books which have food themes.

Work on developing a good relationship between the child and feeder which will help the child trust and respond to the feeder.

12 ·· **Respond calmly** to TBR and jaw clenching. Tension and overreaction in the feeder can contribute to tension in the child. Explore the regular feeder's reactions to the pattern. Panic? Frustration? Anxiety? Is the child aware of these reactions? Is the pattern functioning in some behavioural way?

Video the feeding session. Afterwards sit down with the feeder and analyse the pattern, paying particular attention to what occurs immediately before and immediately after the clenching or tonic bite.

Use the 'Communication Behaviours' checklist on page 22 to help evaluate this area.

Jaw instability overview

An unstable jaw means excessive movement during feeding, so that there is no stable base for the movement of other structures (eg. tongue) involved in the feeding process. Jaw elevation does not occur, resulting in problems with sucking and chewing. In infants who are breast-fed, the jaw makes wider excursions than in bottle-fed babies. Cup drinking has different requirements from bottle drinking as greater jaw stability is required.

Normal Development

Internal jaw stability develops from age 18 to 24 months (Winstock, 1994). Prior to this, external stability may be achieved, for example, by biting the rim of a cup. Alexander (1987) notes this occurring from age 13 to 15 months.

Causes and Contributory Factors

Premature infants who have poorly developed tone and bulk in the orofacial area may suffer from jaw instability. Other possible causes or contributory factors are neck hyperextension, abnormal tongue movements and orofacial hypotonia or facial paresis (weakness) (Wolf and Glass, 1992).

Additionally, jaw instability can be a stress reaction, particularly in the child whose neurological state is poor.

Therapy guidelines

1 ⋯ **Correct positioning** is important. Head and neck alignment is the key to treating excessive jaw movement. Use a position with the head in neutral alignment or in slight flexion. With some children, extreme chin tuck, where the chin should be close to the chest, may help. This will provide support. To be effective, the head must be held very stable – to maintain this position, an angled neck bottle may be useful.

The infant's breathing must always be monitored, as extreme neck flexion may produce airway obstruction, particularly in cases where neck hyperextension is necessary to maintain an airway.

2 ⋯ **Focus on the main problem area.** Concentrate on the appropriate structure or function, for example, tongue movement or hypotonia. See relevant sections/chapters.

3 ⋯ **Provide external support** to encourage jaw stability in preparation for the food. Use firm pressure of the finger under the jaw. Wolf and Glass (1992) recommend that, with this position, the bottle or cup is held between the thumb and index fingers while upward pressure is provided to the mandible by the third and fourth fingers.

Use two fingers, one on the chin and the other under the chin, when feeding from the side.

Stand behind the child and support his jaw with the palm of one hand. Tip the cup with the other hand. If necessary, support the child's lower lip with the index finger of the hand supporting the jaw.

When feeding from the front, the thumb can be placed on the child's chin, with the index finger facilitating upward movement of the TMJ.

Avoid pressure to the base of the tongue as this can interfere with sucking.

Use a cup or drinking utensil with a weighted base (Winstock, 1994). Evans-Morris and Dunn-Klein (1987) recommend attaching a strap to go around the chin to a hat or cap and encouraging the child to wear it when drinking. It must not be so tight that the jaw remains closed, but must be tight enough to assist with elevation and closure by providing resistance.

4 · · · **Encourage internal stability.** Reduce external support as the child develops internal stability. Regularly remove external support to assess whether it is still required and reduce its use as appropriate. With cup drinking, encourage the child to hold the cup edge with his teeth unless a tonic bite reflex is present. Maintain as much continual contact between the cup and lower lip as possible. Do not keep removing it, even when the child stops drinking (Evans-Morris and Dunn-Klein, 1987).

Too small a bolus may not provide enough stimulation for jaw movement and control. Experiment with bigger boluses.

5 · · · **Work on lip closure.** Give direct support to the cheeks and lips or the lower lip if the child is hypotonic. Ensure a good latch. Develop oro-motor control with blowing and sucking activities. Use candles, bubbles and straws where appropriate. See 'Lip Seal' guidelines on pages 61–63.

6 · · · **Eliminate practices which may contribute to jaw instability.** Too small a food portion may not provide enough stimulus for mouth closure and jaw stability. Try bigger boluses.

Do not remove spoon rapidly, as this will affect internal stability and control.

Do not scrape food off the child's dental ridge when removing the spoon, as this will contribute to an extension and open mouth pattern.

Do not present food or utensils rapidly. Alert the child to their presentation verbally and visually and keep the speed with which they are introduced consistent and predictable. Establishing a rhythm will help with internal control.

7 · · · **Normalize sensation.** Tapping and stroking around the muscles of the jaw and the TMJ can facilitate appropriate jaw action. Play games such as patty cake and peek-a-boo (Evans-Morris and Dunn-Klein, 1987; Wolf and Glass, 1992).

8 · · · **Demonstrate a stable and steady mouth** outside and within the feeding session. This will provide the child with a good model.

Jaw thrust overview

Jaw thrust can be quite sudden, forceful and exaggerated. Alexander (1987) describes it as 'a strong depression of the lower jaw' with a 'force greater than that seen in normal sucking'. The jaw may become stuck in the open position and abnormal patterns such as head and neck hyperextension may be reinforced.

58

Causes and Contributory Factors

According to Wolf and Glass (1992), jaw thrust may be associated with dislocation of the tempero mandibular joint (TMJ) or cervical spine, infected or painful teeth or gums, neck hyperextension and hypersensitivity.

Classification

Alexander (1987) classifies jaw thrust into two main types: (1) jaw thrust with tongue protrusion and forward pushing of the lower jaw (this is a compensatory movement in an attempt to stabilize the jaw); and (2) jaw thrust with tongue retraction and backward movement of the jaw (this pattern is initially seen with head and neck hyperextension).

Therapy guidelines

1 ··· **Consult medical or dental staff** to rule out complications.

2 ··· Prior to feeding, **provide preparatory handling**, which can help stabilize and reduce hypertonia and extension patterns. Reduce tone through rocking, calming music and so on.

Place the child prone on the feeder's lap or wedge before feeding. Gravity will help the jaw move forward naturally (Evans-Morris and Dunn-Klein, 1987). A hand placed under the jaw and moved forward will provide slight traction, which may help *(ibid)*. Ensure that the child does not respond to this approach with resistance, resulting in increased tension.

3 ··· **Provide jaw stability** where appropriate. See 'Jaw Instability' guidelines, above.

4 ··· **Position the child appropriately**, particularly where extension is present. Encourage a flexed pattern including neck elongation and body and head alignment. Evaluate how much maintaining an airway is dependent on neck hyperextension, as this will have implications for positioning.

5 ··· **Reduce environmental stimuli** so that the child can concentrate on feeding. This is particularly important with hypertonia and with children with a poor neurological state. Remove auditory stimuli, for example by turning off the television. Reduce visual stimuli such as bright lights or direct sunlight. Remove combined stimuli such as the presence of extra people. See 'Child Preparation' guidelines (pages 92–94).

6 ··· **Work on desensitization and normalization.**

Use a toothbrush (for gums, teeth, cheek and tongue).

Use rubber toys with appendages, the child's or the feeder's fingers for mouthing practice.

Rub outside and on the surface of gum ridges. Use a variety of textures, such as a washcloth, or cotton wool (moistened to ensure that it does not come apart in the child's mouth).

Gradually introduce a range of different tastes, increasing the range as the child copes better. For example, experiment with sweet and sour foods. A non-nutritive example provided by Wolf and Glass (1992) is the use of toothpaste with the toothbrush (the child's mouth can be cleaned with a syringe).

Increasing the range of consistencies if this is appropriate to the child.

See 'Orofacial Hypersensitivity' guidelines (pages 74–77).

7 · · · Help the child to **experience a closed mouth sensation**, initially outside and then during a feeding session. The thumb can be placed either on the child's TMJ or under the lower lip, with the rest of the hand supporting the jaw. Gently facilitate a closed mouth. Evans-Morris and Dunn-Klein (1987) recommend play activities such as holding a cloth between the teeth and shaking it in imitation of a dog. Demonstrate this first, then encourage the child to copy if appropriate. Firm but gentle tapping around the TMJ should help with appropriate movement and patterns *(ibid)*. See 'Lip Seal' guidelines (pages 61–63).

8 · · · **Reduce stimulation that may contribute to the pattern.** For example, use a narrower spoon and smaller bolus.

Lip seal overview

Function and Effects

The tongue, cheeks and lips work closely together to achieve lip seal. Poor lip seal may lead to excessive dribbling or excessive liquid or food loss during feeding with implications for nutritional intake if severe. When the lip seal is intermittently broken with bottle-fed children, a smacking sound will accompany this loss of suction.

Normal Development

At age six months, the lower lip can protrude independently under a cup or spoon to provide stability (Alexander, 1987). The upper lip is active in removing food from the spoon by age nine to 12 months, and making a seal when drinking from age 12 to 18 months (Winstock, 1994). By age 18 months, the child can chew with lips closed and by 24 months he can lip seal when drinking. This skill gradually develops until by three to four years of age, lip closure is complete during feeding.

Causes and Contributory Factors

Problems can result from (1) orofacial hypotonia where the mouth is consistently open; (2) reduced cheek stability including diminished sucking pads in young infants; (3) jaw instability, which will affect the child's ability to create and maintain a continual lip seal; (4) jaw thrust, where the jaw is stuck in the open position; (5) conditions where the child is mainly dependent on the oral airway for breathing; (6) tongue protrusion or thrust which will affect the child's ability to establish and preserve lip seal; and (7) the myopathies where an open mouth posture is chronically present.

Therapy guidelines

1 ··· **Treat underlying problems.** Reduced lip seal may result from a number of conditions as outlined above. Treatment should begin at this point. (See 'Orofacial Hypotonia', 'Cheek Stability', 'Jaw Instability', 'Jaw Thrust' or 'Tongue-thrust' guidelines as relevant.)

2 ··· **Ensure flexion** – neck elongation and chin tuck – which will help the lips to be more active in suction or food removal.

61

3 ⋯ **Provide external support.** Support to the cheeks and lips may help increase lip approximation around the teat or spoon. Place the thumb and index finger on the cheeks and facilitate lip pursing (Wolf and Glass, 1992). If the lower lip is hypotonic, support it with a finger. Support the jaw if necessary. Wolf and Glass (1992) recommend using a small bottle which can be supported between the thumb and index finger, leaving the other fingers free for support.

4 ⋯ With bottle-fed children, if sucking activity is observed but intake is minimal, **ensure that a good latch** is achieved. Check that the lower lip is curled outwards. Ensure that the lips approximate the fatter base of the teat. Facilitate this directly if necessary. Try different teats.

5 ⋯ **Provide sensory input** as lip closure is strongly influenced by this. With breast-fed babies, nipple shields may help with the latch, particularly in the initial moments. The increased sensory information may help the development of a more mature pattern. Try different teats to see which is most suitable for the child. Too wide or large a teat may contribute to poor seal by causing excessive mouth opening. However, narrower teats sometimes make seal difficult as the sensory feedback is reduced. Short teats may not provide sufficient stimulation for the adequate closure necessary for active sucking.

Provide larger portions. Evans-Morris and Dunn-Klein (1987) note that the child is more likely to close his lips during chewing if given a larger mouthful and if the food is apt to fall out. With small portions, lip seal may not be necessary. Ensure that the child is not respiratorially compromised when giving a larger bolus.

▼ **Allow some degree of sloppiness by leaving food on the lips both during and after feeding and encouraging the child to remove or clean the food from the labial area** *(ibid)*. **This will also encourage the child's active participation in the process of feeding.**

6 ⋯ **Encourage appropriate lip posturing in readiness for food.** Ensure a flexed position. Place the fingers on the child's cheeks and draw them forward. With one finger, stroke downwards from his nose to the top lip.

Provide firm but gentle circular dabbing around the outside of his lips. Place the food or liquid around or on the lips initially.

Play games, such as patting or peek-a-boo, that involve tapping and patting the TMJ and jaw muscles.

7 ··· With spoon feeding, **give time for lip activity**. Rapid removal of the spoon means that the child may not have time to bring the top lip down to remove food from the spoon. Evans-Morris and Dunn-Klein (1987) recommend that the spoon be presented slowly so that internal stability can be achieved. This will give the child time to organize food removal.

Do not scrape the spoon against the dental ridge or gum when removing it. This practice will not encourage the development of appropriate lip activity and will encourage or contribute to extension patterns.

8 ··· Evans-Morris and Dunn-Klein (1987) and Winstock (1994) recommend that the feeder **present the food at a lower level** than the child's mouth: a higher-level presentation will encourage extension and an open mouth, making lip seal more difficult.

9 ··· **Provide cold stimulation.** Sucking (not licking) on cold and long foods such as frozen lollipops or juice sticks, refrigerated slices of fruit or liquorice sticks will aid closure. Make this more difficult by reducing the size of objects presented. Provide food at an appropriate temperature: food which is too hot will encourage an open mouth response.

10 ·· **Develop oro-motor skills** to help lip control and strength. (Play blowing games.)

▼ **Use candles, bubbles, whistles, pin wheels, or football games using packing material or light tissue paper rolled into small balls and so on.**
▼ **Demonstrate the pattern, using exaggerated lip movements. Using a mirror may help with reinforcement.**
▼ **Initially, have the object as near as is safely possible to the child's lips.**
▼ **Increase the distance as lip strength develops.**

Straws may be used if appropriate.
▼ **Use squeeze bottle drinks initially: they are easier to suck from.**
▼ **Use liquids of different consistencies: thin (water) to thick (milkshakes).**
▼ **Use a range of tastes for enjoyment, reinforcement and increasing sensation. Play guessing games by disguising the contents. Encourage the child to guess what the liquid is.**
▼ **Use a variety of straws. Vary the width (thin to thick), length (short to long) and shape.**

63

Lack of spontaneous mouth opening overview

Normal Development

The rooting reflex, which is characterized by searching movements for the nipple or teat, usually occurs up to age four to five months in the infant. It occurs in response to tactile stimulation on the cheeks or lips and is distinguished by the child's head turning towards the stimulus, and associated mouth opening.

Causes and Contributory Factors

Lack of spontaneous mouth opening most commonly occurs in premature infants. General and orofacial hypotonia may also be responsible. It is observed where states of alertness or neurological insult affect the rapidity with which a child responds to tactile input and opens the mouth.

Therapy guidelines

1 ··· **Encourage the rooting reflex.** Provide tactile stimulation using the teat, nipple or fingers on the cheeks and labial area. Present the teat or nipple while making it easier for the child's head to turn towards it. Insert the teat or nipple gently into the oral cavity.

2 ··· **Provide preparatory handling,** over the whole body or limited to the facial and oral areas to increase tone before the feeding session. Activities include rhythmical rocking or bouncing and so on. See 'Child Preparation' guidelines (pages 92–94).

3 ··· **Focus on increasing tone and sensation** where appropriate. This should improve stability and control.

▼ Work directly on orofacial tone of the cheeks and the area around the lips. Use firm but gentle and fast, rhythmical tapping, vibration and stretching movements over the cheeks and jaw muscles.
▼ Introduce and grade changes according to the child's ability.
▼ Do these activities consistently (about five times a day) for five to 10 minutes (depending on the child's ability to cope) for effects to be noticed.
▼ With breast-fed babies, nipple shields may provide increased sensory input.
▼ Consult a paediatric physiotherapist to help build overall body tone.
▼ See 'Orofacial Hypotonia' guidelines (pages 79–81).

4 · · · **Provide appropriate positioning** to improve internal organization and provide stability and support for movement of the jaw.

- ▼ With hypotonia, the general rule is to position the child in such a way as to encourage flexion which will help with appropriate lip posturing.
- ▼ With low-tone babies or small children, a side-lying position on the feeder's lap with the trunk straight should be of benefit.
- ▼ With children with unstable neurological states, containment, including swaddling, may help internal organization to enable the child to open his mouth.
- ▼ See 'Positioning' guidelines (pages 82–83).

5 · · · **Facilitate jaw movement.** Tap, using fast, gentle but firm movements on the TMJ. Push the chin up slightly with a finger. Provide a wipe movement from the TMJ to the lips. Place the thumb on the bony part of the chin or TMJ and provide gentle but firm pressure.

6 · · · **Encourage appropriate lip posturing in readiness for food.**

- ▼ Ensure a flexed position.
- ▼ Place the fingers on the child's cheeks and draw the lips forward.
- ▼ With one finger, stroke downwards from his nose to the top lip.
- ▼ Provide firm but gentle circular dabbing around the outside of his lips.
- ▼ Place the food or liquid around or on the lips.

Play games, such as patting and peek-a-boo, that involve tapping and patting the TMJ and jaw muscles.

7 · · · **Encourage spontaneous mouth opening.**

- ▼ Make sure that the teat is large enough to stimulate an opening response.
- ▼ Elicit the rooting reflex.
- ▼ Stimulate the lower lip by placing one or two drops of liquid on to it. Alternatively, wet a finger and rub it on the lower lip.

8 · · · **Use rhythm, consistency and routine** to help the child predict and control movements.

65

Overview

Children who present with multiple impairment have a number of modalities affected, for example, sight, hearing, motor skills and so on. There are varying degrees of handicap within this definition, ranging from profound deficits to mild problems. In recent years, because of improved survival rates and medical and technological advances, a greater number of profound, multiply learning disabled (PMLD) children are being referred to the professions. There are obvious implications for the development of feeding skills within this group.

Therapy guidelines

1 · · · **Consistency** is the keyword. Evans-Morris and Dunn-Klein (1987) and Winstock (1994) argue that children with multiple or visual handicaps must know what to expect and when. This increases the child's feeling of control, and actual control over feeding. Develop a routine the child can depend upon. Have the same feeder (particularly important in nursery settings), same utensils, same cues, same rhythm to the feed and the same time each day.

2 · · · **Give the child cues** (signal the production or placement of food, utensils, people). This strategy helps the child predict what happens next and increases participation and feelings of control (Winstock, 1994). It can occur on a number of levels: verbal ("open your mouth", "here comes the spoon"); auditory (tapping the spoon on the plate); visual (presentation of the object); through smell (present the food under the child's nose before feeding); through touch (facilitate tactile exploration of the utensil or food). The feeder can also develop a specific touch-cueing system, if appropriate, to signal changes occurring in the feeding process. For example, a tap on the shoulder, if used consistently by the feeder and just before the presentation of food, could gain meaning for the child to help him understand that the food is coming.

3 ··· **Reduce environmental stimuli** to help the child respond to cues, learn the routine, organize internally and concentrate. The child may have reduced ability to filter out background noise and light. Reduce auditory stimuli (for example, turn off the television); reduce visual stimuli, such as bright lights or direct sunlight, where appropriate; reduce combined stimuli such as the presence of extra people. As the child develops and can cope with more stimuli, reintroduce them selectively and gradually.

4 ··· **Make use of the child's strengths and abilities,** whether these are physical, visual, communicative, auditory or proprioceptive, to encourage his participation in and control of the process. For example, place utensils where he can locate them easily by touch if blind, or where residual vision can pick them out. Also use intact faculties such as smell to interest the child. Be aware of hypersensitivities, such as to touch, taste or smell.

5 ··· With a visually impaired child, Winstock (1994) recommends the **use of contrasts** such as bright, uniform utensils against a dark background (such as a tray, wedge or non–slip mat) to help the child locate items with greater ease.

6 ··· When moving to self-feeding, facilitate the child's participation and control by **providing physical support** at the wrist, elbow or shoulder. These physical prompts and support techniques can be gradually lessened and removed as the child develops.

7 ··· **Familiarize the child with the utensils** involved in feeding through play (Winstock, 1994). Organize 'pretend' play activities with dolls, teddy bears and utensils and food. Play feeding games, including the child and feeder in the activity.

8 ··· Don't rush. The feeder will need to **allocate extra time** for feeding a multiply impaired child.

9 ··· Evans-Morris and Dunn-Klein (1987) caution the clinician to be sensitive to **temperature and food preferences**. If there is a change in the temperature of the taste of food presented, it is important to let the child know in advance by telling, using touch cues, sound effects or facial expressions and so on.

10 ·· Help the feeder to read and **learn the child's communication signals** and reactions. This will help the feeder to understand the child's likes and dislikes, whether they are full or want more, to anticipate problems and to help the child become an active communicator (see the 'Stress Behaviours' checklist [page 20] or the 'Communication Behaviours' checklist [page 22] for detailed analysis). Child communications should always be acknowledged verbally.

67

Overview

The quantity of food consumed by a child depends on a number of factors: the child's size and weight; the child's appetite; the child's medical condition and history; use of supplementary measures, including tube feeding; cultural feeding patterns; the quantity fed to the child; and the frequency with which the child is fed. Frequently fed babies will usually take less than children who are fed at longer time intervals.

Normal Development

Evans-Morris and Dunn-Klein (1987) give an outline of nutritional needs: up to age one month, intake is usually in the order of 2–6 ounces of liquid per six feeds/day; at age three months this has increased to 8 ounces of liquid per four to six feeds/day; at age five months, the child usually has 9–10 ounces of food and liquid per four to six feeds/day; and at age seven months, the child usually has 11 ounces of food and liquid per four to six feeds/day.

Causes and Contributory Factors for Reduced Intake

Preterm children have increased energy requirements due to increased work of breathing, maintenance of normal temperatures and necessary catch-up growth (Neal, 1995). Intake is insufficient for their purposes. Factors which contribute to reduced intake include significant limiting oro-motor and motor patterns; orofacial hypersensitivity, if severe; conditions of significant respiratory compromise; conditions of reduced endurance; unstable neurological states; metabolic disorders and significant food refusal. Significant reflux and/or aspiration can affect the child's tolerance of feeding, cause respiratory problems which also affect the child's feeding and reduce the maintenance of food in the stomach.

The Food Diary

In order to evaluate the child's nutritional intake, the child will need to have his weight regularly monitored and to be seen by a paediatric dietician. The clinician can also use a food diary to help estimate the child's intake and the food consistencies offered or given. The feeder should be sent a copy of the food diary on page 71 and a sample diary, before seeing the child. The diary can also be used to evaluate progress in feeding. To help in converting grams to ounces (weight) and millilitres to ounces (capacity), use the following chart.

WEIGHT	CAPACITY
1 gram = 0.035 ounces	*1 millilitre = 0.035 ounces*
62.5 grams = 2.187 ounces	*62.5 millilitres = 2.187 ounces*
125 grams = 4.375 ounces	*125 millilitres = 4.375 ounces*
1 kilogram = 2.2 pounds	*1 litre = 1.76 pints*

SAMPLE FOOD DIARY

NAME David Power

DAY Friday

DATE 8th February

TIME FED	LOCATION/ SEATING USED	FOOD/DRINK DESCRIPTIONS	AMOUNT OFFERED	AMOUNT TAKEN	WHO FED CHILD	HOW LONG IT TOOK	WHO WAS PRESENT
7.00 am	In Mum's bed	Bottle of formula	8 oz	Nil	David by himself	15 minutes	Mum
9.30 am	In the kitchen in his high chair	Porridge with full cream milk	2 oz of porridge and 4 oz of milk	About half	Mum with David helping	30 minutes	Mum
10.30 am	Around the house while playing	Blackcurrant drink	4 oz	All	David	On and off until lunchtime	David and sometimes Mum
12.00 noon	In the kitchen in his high chair	Jar of chicken and vegetable dinner and yogurt	4 oz jar and 75g pot	None of the dinner and all of the yogurt	Mum	40 minutes	Mum and neighbour's child
1.00 pm	In his bed	Bottle of formula	8 oz	All	David	15 minutes	David only
3.30 pm	In the main room while watching television	Blackcurrant drink and chocolate biscuits	4 oz of drink and 2 biscuits	All the drink and both biscuits	David	On and off until dinner time	Older sisters
6.00 pm	In the kitchen in his high chair	Beefburger, mashed potatoes and peas	1 burger, 3 tblsp of potatoes and 1 tsp of peas	None of the burger or peas, 2 tsp of potato	Mum and oldest sister	One hour	Mum, Dad and two older sisters
7.30 pm	In his bed	Bottle of formula	8 oz	6 oz (fell asleep)	David	15 minutes	Mum

THE MANUAL OF PAEDIATRIC FEEDING PRACTICE

FOOD DIARY

NAME

DATE

DAY

TIME FED	LOCATION/ SEATING USED	FOOD/DRINK DESCRIPTIONS	AMOUNT OFFERED	AMOUNT TAKEN	WHO FED CHILD	HOW LONG IT TOOK	WHO WAS PRESENT

Explanatory note for feeder

In order to help with feeding difficulties, it is important to know what your child usually has to eat and drink. Please fill in the 'Food Diary' for three days, preferably including a Saturday or Sunday. A sample diary is provided to help you.

Use household measures, such as slices, teaspoons or tablespoons, and container sizes, such as 4 ounce jar of baby food, 125 gram pot of yogurt, or 6 ounce bottle.

71

Therapy guidelines

1 · · · **Consider tube feeding**, particularly where there is significant aspiration, failure to thrive, or significant dehydration.

Where tube feeding is short-term, nasogastric tubes are sufficient. Where it is long-term, gastro tube feeding is more appropriate as aversive behaviours can develop in the orofacial area from use of naso or orogastric tubes and the practices that surround them, such as cleaning and reinsertion. Additionally, breathing can be compromised in children with respiratory and congestion problems.

2 · · · **Refer to a paediatric dietician**, who may advise on commercial supplements and general nutrition.

3 · · · **Increase the fat content** of the diet. This should be done under the guidance and approval of the paediatric dietician. When changing a child's diet, it is important to consider his age and to be alert for any signs or symptoms that may indicate an allergic reaction, or may contribute to current problems such as reflux or aspiration. Winstock (1994) makes the following suggestions, which are particularly suitable for children over 12 months of age:

▼ Add cream to pudding, potatoes, cereals and so on.
▼ Add butter to potatoes and so on.
▼ Fry food whenever possible.
▼ Melt chocolate into puddings and drinks.
▼ Add cheese to sauces and potatoes.
▼ Use cheese with a high fat content, such as cream cheese and cheddar.
▼ Add smooth peanut butter to vegetables.
▼ Include pastry where suitable.
▼ Use fortified milk for older children. Add two tablespoons of skimmed milk powder to a pint of whole milk.
▼ Use snacks. Monitor to see if a child becomes too full to eat main meals.

4 · · · **Conserve the child's energy** before, during and after feeding. Do not bathe, dress or play with the child before or just after feeding. With children with reduced endurance or respiratory compromise, provide rests halfway through feeding to ensure that energy expenditure does not outweigh the nutritional intake.

5 · · · **Position the child appropriately** to increase control, stability and the benefits from feeding (Alexander, 1987). See 'Positioning' guidelines (pages 82–83).

6 ··· **Ensure that practices are conducive to good nutritional intake.** This includes consideration of the utensils and textures used.

7 ··· If the child is feeding orally but still has a tube in place, **supplement oral intake with overnight tube feeds**. Be careful, however, not to overfeed, so that the child continues to be motivated to feed orally.

8 ··· **Use consistent feeders.**

9 ··· **Try demand feeding** (feeding when the child is hungry) with young infants who may be motivated to take more food if fed in this manner.

10 ·· Continue to **monitor weight** through liaison with the paediatric dietician and health visitor.

11 ·· **Reduce parental concerns.** Many feeders are so concerned with ensuring that the child receives adequate nutrition that other concerns and recommended practice can sometimes be neglected. Provide rationales for recommendations. Continually reinforce recommendations. Ensure regular weight monitoring and advice on nutrition through health visitors and paediatric dieticians. Consider referring the parents for support and counselling.

Overview

Hypersensitive or aversive responses are increased sensation to touch. They are stronger than normal reactions and are out of proportion to the stimulus. Reduced responses result from decreased sensation to touch. The ability to discriminate the sensory input appropriately is impaired.

These responses are most commonly associated with touch and may be limited to tactile input; alternatively, they may include a number of areas, such as taste, temperature and smell.

Causes and Contributory Factors

These conditions may arise for a number of reasons. Premature babies may have an immature neurological development. They may be children with poor neurological states, or who have a history of negative oral experiences and aversive stimuli such as tube feeding, suctioning and intubation. With children who are chronically ill, their resources are mainly focused on survival and there is therefore reduced ability to manage sensory input. Delays in the introduction of oral feeding (not just liquids, but solids and cup drinking) can mar the child's reactions if the critical or sensitive period when introduction normally occurs is missed (Wolf and Glass, 1992). Children with abnormal postural tone and movement development may have developed a base of abnormal sensation (Alexander, 1987).

Therapy guidelines

1 ⋯ **Positioning** of the child should ensure comfort and stability, with the emphasis on an upright position, flexion and symmetry. This will help with internal organization. See 'Positioning' guidelines (pages 82–83).

2 ⋯ **Preparatory handling** will help the child integrate sensory information and build up tolerance. Handling should be firm but sensitive and graded according to the child's abilities and coping responses. Handling is important throughout the day and before feeding. Examples of general handling are patting the head, hugging, rocking, holding, walking up and down stairs, and swinging. Play slow music, gradually increasing the rhythm (Winstock, 1994). Practise reduction in environmental stimuli, with gradual and graded reintroduction. Focus on improving concentration skills. Massage should also be considered, where appropriate. See 'Child Preparation' guidelines (pages 92–94) for more details.

74

3 ⋯ **Reduce environmental stimuli** which may contribute to the child's disorganization and reduce concentration on the feeding process. These include auditory stimuli, such as television and radio; visual stimuli, such as bright lights and direct sunlight; and combined stimuli, such as the presence of extra people.

4 ⋯ **Reduce aversive orofacial stimuli** as much as possible by evaluating care routines and the child's response to them. For example, where appropriate, modify or eliminate activities such as suctioning, use of a nasogastric tube, frequent removal and reinsertion of naso- or orogastric tubes, and change taping procedures; also, where appropriate, a gastrostomy should be considered as an alternative for prolonged nasogastric tube feeding, which may help to reduce the level of current aversive stimuli.

5 ⋯ **Eliminate utensils which may contribute to the hypersensitivity.** A long teat will elicit the gag reflex more easily than a short teat. With a child who is oversensitive to the teat, use of a medicine cup may help feeding.

6 ⋯ Even with non-orally fed children, **develop the non-nutritive suck** (NNS). This will help in maintaining and developing oral skills and an understanding of the link between the mouth and stomach. Use a teat blocked with moistened gauze, which will decrease air intake initially, to see how the child copes with increased saliva production: the feeder can then experiment with different shapes and sizes. Then use a dummy/pacifier.

7 ⋯ **Focus on specific problem areas** where necessary. For example, where gagging is evident, work on reducing this response.

8 ⋯ **Provide orofacial exploration and stimulation.** Many children with feeding and motor or sensory difficulties may have reduced or negative experiences in this area. A programme for sensory normalization can use a number of sensory modalities.

▼ **Always begin outside the feeding sessions in the initial period.**
▼ **Provide grading of stimuli. Begin in the range where the child is comfortable and used to having contact. Build up to the point where the stimulus is not tolerated, backtracking slightly at signs of increased intolerance, tone, anxiety or stress.**
▼ **Go slowly to help the child adapt and become accustomed to the stimuli.**
▼ **Monitor the child's responses through changes in the autonomic, motoric and state-related behaviours. If stress behaviour surfaces, lower the intensity of stimuli (Brodsky, 1993).**
▼ **Practise this for short periods, five to eight times a day.**
▼ **Stimuli should be symmetrical (Winstock, 1994).**

75

▼ Stimuli should be presented from proximal (furthest point) to distal (nearest point): for example, fingers → arms → neck → chin → cheeks → lips → gum → tongue. Move on to more distal areas once tolerance in one place has developed. For example, from the neck, move to the back of the head, to the crown, the forehead, cheeks and so on.

▼ The type of tactile stimulation can also be graded. Texture usually goes from the smooth to soft to unusual or prickly; pressure along a continuum from light to firm.

▼ When working on mouthing, start by using the feeder's finger, the child's fingers or hands if physically possible, toothbrush or toothbrush trainer, identifying parts as they are touched.

▼ The child should be encouraged to suck on a number of items – variety is important – as he should not get attached to only one item, which will limit his abilities.

▼ When working orally, care should be taken to avoid frequent stimulation of the gag response.

▼ The use of a mirror will help the child to be more aware of, and comfortable with, himself (Wolf and Glass, 1992).

▼ Hypersensitive children appear to have greater tolerances for smooth textures, firm pressure and puréed foods. Individual children vary and experimenting outside the continuum may be valuable for progress.

9 ⋯ **Develop the range of tastes and textures** available to the child as appropriate.

Food textures go thus: liquid → puréed → untextured chunky → crunchy. Make graded changes as the child is able to cope with them. For some children with swallowing and breathing problems, a small reverse in this sequence may be advisable. For example, where a child is unable to cope with a liquid consistency, try puréed food. As the child comes to tolerate this, thin out the purée to a thick liquid, and then a thin liquid.

Gradually introduce changes in texture, smell, taste and temperature. Do not introduce too many changes at once which may contribute to hypersensitivity.

10 ⋯ **Use of firm touch and pressure,** which is known to have an integrating effect on the central nervous system, can be provided in a number of ways:

▼ Rubbing the body with various textures (hands, washcloth, brush, stuffed toys, cloths such as cotton, silk, corduroy and so on).

▼ **Rubbing the gums or stroking the tongue. Provide firm pressure to the outer gum ridge starting at the midline and travelling to the back of the gums. Repeat three or four times on each side of the lower and upper gums, with pauses between upper and lower to allow the child to swallow saliva.**

▼ **Touch or pressure can be provided throughout the day through bathing (towelling, moisturizing) and dressing.**

▼ **Vibration through small, hand-held vibrators or finger-tips may be useful. Vibration can be directed to specific areas.**

▼ **Massage should also be considered, where appropriate.**

11 ·· **Encourage a playful and relaxed attitude towards feeding and the orofacial area.** Where appropriate, let the child play with messy (puréed) food on a plastic mat or in a plastic bath. Do 'pretend' play activities using utensils and dolls, teddies and so on. Encourage the child to feed the toys and the feeder. Provide an environment of mutual exploration between the feeder's and child's mouths. Activities may include counting teeth, comparing structures and functions, hiding appropriate food or searching for imaginary toys (Arvedson, 1993b). Tell happy stories or read books with food themes.

12 ·· Where appropriate, **use visual imaging and positive thinking.** These activities should be employed outside the feeding session initially, then before feeding, and finally, as the child copes better, within the session. Use appropriate videos to help the child become calm and relaxed; use calming music; tell stories about pleasant feeding experiences such as picnics and on the beach (Evans-Morris and Dunn-Klein, 1987). Encourage the feeder to visualize successful feeding. Make sure the feeder focuses on the child.

13 ·· The carer should always **use verbal cues** to guide the child through activities and particularly to introduce new objects and sensations.

14 ·· Help the feeder to **read the child's communication signals**, which can help to anticipate problems or to indicate distress or lack of comfort. See the 'Stress Behaviours' checklist (page 20) or the 'Communication Behaviours' checklist (page 22) for a detailed analysis.

15 ·· **Use touch** when communicating with the child during the day (Evans-Morris and Dunn-Klein, 1987).

16 ·· **Integrate treatment into daily routines.** In addition to these activities occurring in preparation for the feeding session, they should be carried out in short, frequent applications. They are often more readily accepted if they occur while the child is attending to something else.

Orofacial hypertonia overview

Increased tone may result in abnormal movement patterns of the tongue, jaw, cheeks and/or lips. Wolf and Glass (1992) note that hypertonia in the orofacial area may eventually lead to abnormal alignment of the orofacial structures. The presence of orofacial hypertonia will significantly affect the success of oral feeding in proportion to its severity.

Causes and Contributory Factors

Wolf and Glass (1992) outline the main factors affecting tone in the orofacial area. They may be part of an overall pattern of hypertonia resulting from a neurological insult or abnormality; a child with an unstable neurological state may respond to a stressful environment or situation (such as feeding) with hypertonic patterns.

Therapy guidelines

1 ··· **Provide preparatory handling** to reduce overall tone and improve general stability and alignment. Place emphasis on the head, neck and shoulders. Try placing the child prone on the feeder's lap before feeding. Evans-Morris and Dunn-Klein (1987) suggest that this technique will encourage relaxation and flexion, which will reduce the potential for hypertonic reactions and patterns. Use general preparation techniques including gentle rocking and bouncing, and calm music to help the child's internal organization and control. Consult the child's paediatric occupational therapist or physiotherapist for specific guidelines.

2 ··· **Provide correct positioning** to help maintain the effects of preparatory handling and to facilitate more appropriate movements of the orofacial structures. The emphasis should be on flexion and support. Most important will be chin tuck (the degree will depend on the individual child) as this position helps reduce the occurrence and effects of orofacial hypertonia. See 'Positioning' guidelines (pages 82–83).

3 ··· **Reduce environmental stimuli.** This lessens the chances of overstimulating the child, which may encourage reduced internal control and stability and contribute to hypertonic patterns. Reducing distracting stimuli will also help the child to concentrate his energies on the feeding process. Reduce auditory stimuli such as the television by turning the volume down, or preferably turning the set off. Remove distracting visual stimuli, such as direct sunlight or bright room lights. Reduce multiple stimuli such as the presence of too many people in the room.

4 ··· **Reduce tone** directly by concentrating on the orofacial area. For example, use the fingers to apply firm but gentle, rhythmical pressure along the target area. Wolf and Glass (1992) recommend the sides of the nose, jaw and mouth, or above and below the lips. They also recommend sandwiching the cheeks between two extended fingers and following this with rapid shaking or vibration, with slight traction.

With hypertonia, the general rule is one of using slow, graded movements when conducting direct work in the orofacial area. This helps the child predict, organize and experience more controlled and less tense sensations and patterns.

5 ··· Encourage the feeder and child to **view the feeding process positively**. Use relaxing videos or calming music before feeding time. Tell stories with positive food themes such as picnics or going to the beach. Help the feeder to visualize successful feeding before the actual feeding of the child (Evans-Morris and Dunn-Klein, 1987).

6 ··· **Reduce or eliminate activities which contribute to hypertonic patterns.** If spoon feeding is being used, encourage the feeder not to remove food by scraping the spoon against the gum or dental ridge. This encourages extension and patterns of hypertonicity: Winstock (1994) recommends that the child be encouraged to use the lips to remove the food. Present food at a slightly lower level than the child's mouth. Higher levels will again encourage extension and hypertonic patterns.

7 ··· **Focus on attention development** with the child through play and general activities.

Orofacial hypotonia overview

Orofacial hypotonia leads to reduced stability and control of the orofacial structures. Response to treatment is dependent on the severity and cause of the hypotonia.

Causes and Contributory Factors

These include generalized hypotonia (for example, Down's syndrome, myopathies) and prematurity, where the child's system may not be mature.

Therapy guidelines

1 ··· **Build overall body tone.** Consult the child's paediatric physiotherapist.

2 ··· **Provide preparatory handling** before the feeding session. This will help promote tone and internal organization.

▼ **Use general handling techniques, such as rocking, bouncing, or the feeder carrying the child while walking up and down the stairs.**
▼ **Direct work to building overall body tone, for example with massage.**
▼ **Consult the child's paediatric physiotherapist.**
▼ **Direct tactile input to the orofacial area. See (4) below.**

3 ··· **Provide appropriate positioning.** Positioning the child correctly will facilitate stability and, consequently, control of the orofacial structures.

▼ **The general rule is one of flexion. Feeding is usually easier when the child is in a flexed position. Individual children will vary, however.**
▼ **Low-tone babies may benefit from lying on their side. Place the child on the feeder's lap facing the feeder, with the trunk straight and well supported. This position encourages flexion and requires less energy expenditure.**
▼ **Where appropriate, try using a standing frame, which should contribute to the normalization of overall tone.**
▼ **Consult the child's paediatric occupational therapist or paediatric physiotherapist.**
▼ **See 'Positioning' guidelines (pages 82–83).**

4 ··· **Improve orofacial tone** and sensory discrimination. Where hypotonia is present, the child will generally require a rapid speed of well-graded stimuli (Alexander, 1987), such as tapping with a finger. Firm tapping or vibration (using fingers or a commercial vibrator) applied directly to the area may increase tone. Grade the quantity of input and the area receiving input. As the child's tolerance develops, increase the amount of input and the area covered. See 'Orofacial Hypersensitivity' guidelines (pages 74–77) for details.

5 ··· **Concentrate on specific problem areas.** The child may present with general problems such as reduced endurance, or difficulties related specifically to hypotonia, such as tongue retraction. See 'Reduced Endurance', 'Tongue Retraction' guidelines and so on where appropriate.

6 ··· **Provide therapy on a frequent and consistent basis.** Work on building tone will only have lasting benefits under these conditions.

▼ **Start building tone directly for a few minutes several times a day.**
▼ **Grade the input for quantity, area covered and frequency of input.**
▼ **Be consistent in application.**
▼ **Provide input during the day and before feeding.**
▼ **Activities to build tone should involve the whole body: consult the paediatric occupational therapist or paediatric physiotherapist.**

7 ··· Where the child's hypotonia affects the ability to suck during feeding, Wolf and Glass (1992) recommend **providing a quick stretch** over the cheek muscles, or on the lips and tongue, during a sucking pause. Make sure that the child does not need this time for breathing, recovery and so on. This technique is best done when the problem is due solely or mainly to hypotonia rather than other factors.

Overview

Correct positioning is vital to the success of oral feeding. As Alexander (1987) notes, it can reduce the influence of abnormal movements, decrease the potential for abnormality and create a base of stability which allows for more functional and fine motor control.

Normal Development

Evans-Morris and Dunn-Klein (1987) give guidelines on the development of positioning in children without difficulties. Up to age three months, children can be fed in a variety of positions, usually whatever is comfortable for the feeder and child; general preferences are for supine, with the head slightly elevated, sidelying, prone on the feeder's chest, or in a semi-supported position. As the child grows and gains in strength and control, the position is more likely to be semi-supported sitting, usually at a 45 to 90 degree angle. From age seven months, children are generally sitting independently. However, they may not be stable and this will place stress on their newly acquired sitting skills. Consequently, extra support is generally required. This is usually provided by a highchair, with a towel at the nape of the neck for additional support. The angle at this stage is normally 90 degrees. By age nine months, internal stability is generally achieved, with the child requiring only a little external support such as a highchair, or a feeder's lap. Independent use of the limbs is developing.

Therapy guidelines

1 ⋯ Consult the child's paediatric occupational therapist.

2 ⋯ **Maintain an overall feeling of flexion** as the general rule. This facilitates a number of oro-motor patterns such as sucking, lip seal and swallowing by increasing the potential for appropriate patterns and control, and by aiding laryngeal closure. A flexed position also helps protect the airway (Wolf and Glass, 1992). Where neck hyperextension is present and functioning to provide an airway, slight extension of the neck can help by increasing the diameter of the pharyngeal airway.

3 ⋯ **Align the head and neck** with the body. Body alignment is characterized by neck elongation with neutral head flexion (Alexander, 1987). The head and extremities should be centred.

4 ⋯ The **shoulders should be symmetric** and forward.

5 ⋯ **Provide support.** Ensure that the head is supported. With infants, this may involve cradling the head, or swaddling. With older children, a towel placed at the nape of the neck when they are seated can help stability. With an older child, the arms can be supported through use of a tray, and, with infants, by the feeder's arm or swaddling. With older children, the feet can be supported by a foot rest or by sturdy, everyday items such as a telephone book. With infants, foot support can be provided through correct positioning by the feeder's body or through techniques such as swaddling.

6 ⋯ **Provide stability.** This can be achieved in a number of ways:

▼ **preparatory handling techniques such as rocking or bouncing to encourage internal control and organization;**

▼ **provision of tactile input to decrease or increase tone or reduce hypersensitivity where appropriate;**

▼ **by providing appropriate support through seating or feeder;**

▼ **appropriate positioning;**

▼ **use of appropriate seating equipment;**

▼ **presentation of food at an appropriate level – the feeder should be positioned at the child's eye level when the child is sitting, and food should be presented slightly below the mouth (presentation at higher levels will encourage extension and abnormal patterns);**

▼ **use of child-facilitated stability, such as the child holding the bottle or cup.**

7 ⋯ **Provide upright positioning** where appropriate. This helps with digestion, facilitates improved oro-motor patterns and reduces the likelihood and effects of reflux and aspiration.

8 ⋯ **Consider the positioning options** available, as outlined in the chart below.

83

OPTIONS

POSITION	FEATURES	USES	CAUTION
Containment	Swaddling the limbs and body through use of a blanket and so on	Containment is useful for children with unstable neurological states and those requiring support. It helps with integration, control and the child's ability to focus on the feeding process	Always monitor the child's signals to see how he is coping with containment and feeding
Supine in lap	The infant or small child is placed supine, facing the feeder, on the feeder's lap, near the feeder's knee	The supine position is good for tube feeding; the feeder is free to use a finger or dummy for non-nutritive sucking, or to facilitate a sucking rhythm	This position does not necessarily help with organization, therefore it may be hard to control side-to-side head movements
Sidelying in lap	The trunk is straight and supported, with the child on the feeder's lap, on his side, facing the feeder	Sidelying helps with flexion generally and specifically, as in tongue retraction; it is useful for hypotonia; it is beneficial for children with reduced endurance as it requires less energy expenditure	The feeder must watch for the head moving into extension
En face	The feeder's feet are placed on a chair opposite her and her knees are drawn up; the child is placed in the feeder's lap facing the feeder, with his head supported by the feeder's legs or hand	This position is useful for small children who hyperextend; the child remains free to turn his head and extend his arms	

POSITION	FEATURES	USES	CAUTION
Standing	A standing frame is the normal method used to achieve this position. Straps may be needed for safety and to ensure stability and posture. Wolf and Glass (1992) recommend that the feet should be well supported with equal weight bearing and the hips should be symmetrical and aligned with the feet. This is the position of greatest body extension which helps to provide stability	Standing is useful with hypotonic children as it inhibits overflexion and normalizes muscle tone (due to gravity). Standing eases the descent of food and therefore may help where reflux and aspiration after the swallow are present	Standing is not a suitable position if it encourages the child to extend. Care should be taken to avoid pressure in the abdominal area which would affect comfort, food digestion, reflux potential, and may encourage extension
Sitting	Right angles are essential at the hips, elbows, knees and ankles (Winstock, 1994; Wolf and Glass, 1992). The seating used should provide good back support (Wolf and Glass, 1992). Arms and feet should be flat and supported by trays and foot rests. Neck and head stability should be ensured with a headrest or towel rolled up and placed at the nape of the neck. Non-slip mats or straps may provide further stability (Winstock, 1994; Wolf and Glass, 1992). The height of the chair and its distance in relation to the tray or table should be considered: too high a tray may result in extension; too low a table may result in overflexion; too close a contact between the chair and table may promote extension (Brodsky, 1993; Evans-Morris and Dunn-Kelin, 1987)	Where stability and support are achieved, sitting helps with flexion and limits abnormal patterns which may affect feeding	Sitting may be unrealistic or require adaptations if head and neck control are a problem. Internal support (child's ability to self support) and external support (from equipment or feeder) are necessary, particularly where the child is expected to feed independently

85

Overview

The introduction of oral feeding to children who have no experience of it can be a difficult and long-term process. Initiating oral feeding with such children should be proceeded with extremely carefully. Oral feeding should not be introduced until the child has reached a gestational age of at least 33 weeks. Although the current trend is to introduce oral feeding earlier and earlier, preterm infants are usually not ready to cope with oral feeding until this age. Additionally, it is wise to err on the side of caution, as aversive behaviours may develop as the direct result of too early an introduction of oral feeding.

Causes and Contributory Factors

Delays in introducing oral feeding can result from a number of factors, such as prematurity, where the child's system is not able to cope with oral feeding when he is born; or the use of tube feeding, where the child has not been able to feed orally for any number of reasons.

When considering whether to introduce oral feeding to an individual child, the clinician must ask a number of questions and base the decision on the answers to these queries as well as the result of clinical probes (see 'Prefeeding Checklist'). With a child who has had no experience of oral feeding, these probes must always be carefully administered, with the child's responses carefully monitored.

The clinician may not be in a position to answer some of the questions posed, unless oral feeding has been attempted. For example, the clinician may not know if aspiration or reflux is present because oral feeding has not been tested and radiological techniques have not been employed. Use of checklists in individual sections, for example 'Clinical Indications of Aspiration' (page 15), will help with regard to particular areas. As far as possible, the clinician should try to answer all the questions posed. Other considerations may arise with regard to the individual child which have not been considered here.

For further analysis, see also the 'Changes of Feeding Method' checklist on page 158. Additionally, because the child's communication signals are important indicators of how the child is coping with oral feeding, use of the 'Stress Behaviours' checklist and the 'Communication Behaviours' checklist is recommended.

PREFEEDING CHECKLIST

NAME	DATE

Stage 1: *Clinical and History Observations*

QUESTION	ANSWER
1 ··· Is aspiration present? If so, is it currently significant enough to prevent or radically affect the success of oral feeding?	
2 ··· Is reflux present? If so, is it significant enough to prevent or radically affect the success of oral feeding?	
3 ··· Is hypersensitivity or desensitization present? If so, is it generalized or specific? To what degree is it present? Does it significantly affect responses to non-nutritive and nutritive stimuli?	
4 ··· Is the child's neurological state stable? Does the child have observable fits? Is there evidence of subclinical fitting (where fits are not readily noticeable eg. blank spells)? Does the neurological state support oral feeding?	
5 ··· Is respiratory status compromised? Does it support the introduction of oral feeding?	
6 ··· Does the child present with reduced endurance? Is it serious enough to have an impact on the effectiveness of oral feeding?	
7 ··· Has the child reached the gestational age (33–36 weeks) and weight (more than 3lb) which would support oral feeding?	
8 ··· Do the short- and long-term prognoses for life and general development support the introduction and potential benefit of an oral feeding programme?	

9 ··· Is the feeder ready for, and committed to, oral feeding?	
10 ·· Has oral feeding been attempted previously? With what results? If stopped, what where the reasons for ceasing oral feeding? How did the child respond to oral feeding attempts?	
11 ·· Are medical conditions or structural abnormalities present which would contraindicate the introduction of oral feeding?	

Stage 2: Probe Observations

PROBE	OBSERVATION
1 ··· Non-nutritive suck Present the child with a dummy/pacifier, blocked teat, or finger. Is the suck present?	
2 ··· Nutritive suck Present the child with liquid (via syringe, in a teat and so on) and observe the suck. Is it present, organized, initiated well, strong and so on?	
3 ··· Swallow reflex Does the child manage his oral secretions? Does he swallow liquid presented orally? How quickly does the swallow occur after liquid is presented?	
4 ··· Amount of liquid While monitoring the child's responses, present him with varying amounts of liquid, starting at half a millilitre and moving backwards or forwards in small steps according to the child's ability to cope	

5 ··· Neurological state Monitor the child's state while the various probes are attempted. Does it remain stable or deteriorate either partially or significantly during feeding? Specify neurological state and stress behaviours	
6 ··· Communication and response behaviours Monitor the child's behaviours and responses before and during feeding. Specify what behaviours occur, paying particular attention to the child's responses to changes made during oral trials, such as increasing the amount of liquid presented	
7 ··· Orofacial structure and function Observe structure and function at rest and during feeding. Are limiting structures or patterns present which would affect the success of oral feeding?	

Stage 3: *Summary Observations*

Area	Supports the introduction of oral feeding	Does not support the current introduction of oral feeding – should be considered at a later stage	Does not support the introduction of oral feeding either in the short term or in the foreseeable long term
Clinical and history observations			
Probe observations			

Therapy guidelines

1 ··· When introducing oral feeding to a child with no or limited experience of it, **err on the side of caution**. Too early an introduction can cause subsequent problems such as aversion to orofacial stimuli or oral feeding. This can make the oral feeding process longer and more complex.

2 ··· When introducing oral feeding, **always monitor the child's signals**, including responses and intentional communication behaviours. Work with the child's system rather than against it, through monitoring of behaviours, which will facilitate oral feeding. Observing the child will help in a number of areas: it helps the feeder to understand the child's behaviour and communication modes, to anticipate problems and to understand how the child is coping with oral feeding or changes made to the feeding process. It also facilitates the child's awareness of himself as an active communicator.

3 ··· **Use a consistent feeder** to help monitor behaviours, to facilitate an understanding of the child's feeding abilities, and for consistency and carry-over of suggestions.

4 ··· **Evaluate whether the child is a disorganized or dysfunctional feeder.** The former is related to immaturity, the latter has a neurological basis. This has implications for management and prognosis.

5 ··· **Reduce environmental stimuli** which may overload the child's system, meaning less internal organization, control and concentration on feeding. Reduce auditory stimuli such as a television by turning the volume down, or preferably off; remove visual stimuli such as direct sunlight or bright room lights; remove combined stimuli such as the presence of extra people.

6 ··· **Use preparatory handling** to help internal organization and control. This will help prepare the child for feeding. Use general activities such as gentle rocking, bouncing and swaddling. See 'Orofacial Hypersensitivity' guidelines (pages 74–77).

7 ··· **Provide appropriate positioning** to promote the success of oral feeding. The general rule is flexion, but individuals' needs vary. Evaluate whether neck hyperextension is necessary to maintain an airway. See 'Positioning' guidelines (pages 82–83).

8 ··· In both children with oral feeding aims, and those for whom oral feeding is not to be implemented, there should be a **focus on normalizing sensation and developing motor skills**. Most of these types of activities can be done even when a child is in an intensive

90

care unit and on a ventilator. Touching and movement should be an everyday part of the child's life, but graded according to his abilities and responses. If the child is tube feeding, touch should be a part of this process to normalize it. Touch should also be used during the day when communicating or interacting with the child.

Work on decreasing or increasing sensation, see 'Orofacial Hypersensitivity/Desensitization' guidelines (pages 74–77).

Work on reducing or building tone, where appropriate, see 'Orofacial Hypertonia' guidelines (pages 78–79) or 'Orofacial Hypotonia' guidelines (pages 79–81).

Consult the child's paediatric occupational therapist or physiotherapist so that general body activities can be addressed.

9 ··· **Provide pleasurable and normal oral experiences.** This can reduce the potential for the development of aversive behaviours and, where oral feeding is not the current goal, can help prepare the child for the demands of oral feeding.

Encourage mouthing on a variety of objects. Start small with one item (for example, a finger) and increase the range as the child is able to cope, including variations in the size, taste, texture and so on. Large rubber toys with appendages are good for mouthing.

Encourage sucking on a non-nutritive level. Use a finger, dummy or teat blocked by moistened gauze (not attached to a bottle). This will prevent air from being swallowed. Simulate a sucking rhythm. Use the same teat for non-nutritive and nutritive sucking in the initial stages.

Where appropriate, provide tasting experiences with minute amounts of liquid or food. Try skimming a dummy or finger over the liquid or food and presenting it to the child. Always monitor the child's responses and ability to handle the food.

10 ·· **Stimulate and assist a swallow** directly, where appropriate. Tap the tip of the tongue and the spot on the hard palate where the tongue normally elevates in swallowing. Repeat as necessary (Evans-Morris and Dunn-Klein, 1987).

Firmly but gently stroke a finger down the child's neck, following the floor of the mouth. As a sucking rhythm emerges, introduce small, carefully measured amounts of liquid to the lips and, when appropriate, to the front of the mouth.

11 ·· **Grade changes slowly**, with the emphasis on monitoring the child's ability to cope with them.

12 ·· **Focus on empowering the feeder and promoting feeder–child bonding.** This is particularly important where the mother and child may have had a traumatic birth, and a subsequent loss of ownership of the child and bonding through hospitalization.

91

Child preparation overview

Some children will need to be facilitated before the feeding session in order to increase the potential for successful feeding. In particular, this applies to children who present with unstable neurological states, multiple and profound disabilities, and young gestational ages. Correct preparatory handling and environmental preparation can contribute significantly to the success of feeding both in the short and the long term. Furthermore, good preparation will increase the child's internal organization, control, confidence and concentration for feeding.

Therapy guidelines

1 ··· **Use strategies to alert the child.** Consider whether it is appropriate to alert the child. Is the child drowsy? Is this a sign of reduced endurance, the need to conserve energy, and perhaps inability to cope with oral feeding? Consider the child's gestational age and therefore the appropriateness of alerting him. Infants do not generally demonstrate spontaneous alerting/arousal until around gestational age 37 weeks, and therefore this strategy may be inappropriate.

Modify the temperature. Cooler temperatures will facilitate alerting. Remove extra covers and clothing. Advise the feeder not to hold the child too closely, as the feeder's body warmth may contribute to sleepiness. Always monitor the child's responses, as uncomfortable temperatures will reduce his ability to concentrate on feeding. Wolf and Glass (1992) recommend that changing the temperature be done with caution where premature infants are concerned, and under the guidance of medical staff.

Use movements such as picking up the child, moving the child into a more upright position, moving the limbs gently, or gentle rocking and bouncing. Changes in rhythm will encourage alerting, so do not maintain a consistent and predictable rhythm.

Energetic music or voice will help alert the child. When using voice, try varying the tone, pitch and animation. Where the child is unstable neurologically, start with softer music, increasing the volume and rhythm as the child's ability to cope progresses.

92

Provide light touch, such as tickling or stroking sensitive areas such as the soles of the feet. Use different textures to further encourage arousal.

Use bright light such as in a well-lit room (Evans-Morris and Dunn-Klein, 1987), but monitor the child's responses as bright light may initially be too extreme, particularly with preterm infants who may feed better at night or in a dark room.

Activities such as bathing and dressing may also have an alerting effect. However, be wary of making the water too warm if bathing the child.

Use combined stimuli, such as movement and touch together.

2 ··· **Use strategies to calm and compose the child** where the child is disorganized, irritable or overstimulated. Modify the temperature by holding the child close to the feeder's body for warmth. Turning up the room heating or adding extra covers or clothing may also help. As with alerting, the clinician and feeder must be aware of the child's comfort level. Temperatures which are uncomfortable will reduce the child's attention on feeding. Temperatures which are too high will cause sleepiness. Again, check with medical staff where appropriate, when changing an infant's temperature.

Reduce environmental stimuli such as excess noise and light. Wolf and Glass (1992) recommend a darkened room. Reducing sensory input will aid internal organization, control and preparation for feeding. This is particularly relevant where the child has frequent startled responses and where the feeder needs to listen to and monitor the child's breathing and swallowing.

Use containment, as in holding or swaddling, which will help control movements. Arms should be in the midline and hips flexed.

Use a predictable rhythm when rocking, bouncing or playing music. This will help the child anticipate and organize.

Any changes made should be made slowly.

Handling should be confident rather than unsure. Wolf and Glass (1992) state that clear handling guides the feeding.

Use distracters such as a rattle or a shiny object. This works well with some hypersensitive children as it removes their tension about feeding. Use of this strategy needs to be tested with individual children, as some will respond with less organization and control when presented with a distracter.

Focus on feeder style. Ensure that the feeder is not rushed or disorganized when preparing feeding or when actually feeding the child. Children are generally extremely sensitive to the feeder's style and emotions.

3 ··· As with clear handling, clear preparation directs the feeding. **Ensure that all food, utensils and equipment are to hand** before commencing feeding. A disorganized session will affect a disorganized or uninterested child's ability to feed successfully.

4 ··· **Provide a predictable routine** which functions as outlined above and also helps the child's internal control:

▼ Food and utensils should be placed where the child can see and anticipate them.
▼ Use consistent feeders, positioning and equipment, where appropriate.
▼ Feed at regular time intervals and predictable times.
▼ Make changes gradual.

5 ··· **Ensure that the feeder is mentally prepared** for feeding.

▼ Give clear guidelines on handling, feeding strategies or techniques, the child's condition and ability to cope, and on changes to be made during feeding.
▼ Do not overload the feeder with unnecessary or excess information.
▼ Be consistent in applying recommendations and reinforcing them.
▼ Wolf and Glass (1992) recommend helping the feeder develop a positive mind-set. This involves visualizing the child, the feeder and feeding as successful. The clinician needs to be realistic but confident when applying this principle.
▼ Ensure that the feeder is as relaxed as possible before feeding.
▼ Ensure that the feeder is prepared and organized, with all the needs to hand before the commencement of feeding. Disorganization will affect feeding and the child and the feeder's feelings about feeding.
▼ Take account of the feeder's needs. For example, if the feeder has a back problem, positioning will need to take account of this in addition to the child's needs.

6 ··· Help the feeder to understand and **learn the child's communication signals**. This will help in anticipating problems, understanding the child's likes and dislikes and so on. Communications from the child should be acknowledged verbally. For help in this process, see the 'Stress Behaviours' checklist (page 20) or the 'Communication Behaviours' checklist (page 22).

Feeder preparation overview

Too often the needs and feelings of the feeder are overlooked when concentrating on the child's specific or general difficulties. The feeder needs to be an important consideration in feeding management as she is intimately involved in the feeding and will have a significant impact on the outcome of any therapeutic intervention.

Therapy guidelines

1 ··· **Ensure the feeder's commitment to and preparation for feeding.** This is particularly relevant where the feeder may have been somewhat disempowered by the unexpectedly early arrival of a child, by a long stay in hospital or by a reduced ability to handle and bond with the child.

2 ··· **Help the feeder to understand the nature of the feeding process,** particularly where the likelihood of its being long-term and gradual is high. Too often, feeders expect rapid change and clinicians do not convey information which makes for more realistic understanding of the process. This includes providing information on specific areas of difficulty. It is the feeder, with support from the clinician and other team members, who will be the one to effect changes in the child's feeding skills.

3 ··· **Demonstrate new techniques** rather than merely explaining them. The feeder will retain and benefit more from demonstration, modelling and visual cues than from verbal instruction only.

4 ··· **Ensure that the feeder is relaxed and confident.** A rushed, disorganized or underconfident feeder communicates this to the child during handling, and this can result in the child becoming disorganized, with reduced control. As Wolf and Glass (1992) state, clear handling guides the feeding.

5 ··· **Encourage the feeder to focus on the child rather than herself;** encourage the feeder to visualize the child and feeding as successful (Wolf and Glass, 1992).

6 ··· **Ensure that items needed are immediately and conveniently available.** This helps with feeder and child organization and preparation, as well as enabling the child to anticipate the food. As this strategy may overexcite some children, it is essential to monitor the child's responses and behaviours.

95

▼

7 ⋯ **Ensure feeder comfort** as much as possible. For example, if the feeder suffers from back problems, positioning will need to take account of her requirements, in addition to the child's.

8 ⋯ **Evaluate the feeder's reactions to the feeding process and specific occurrences** such as gagging. This will help to evaluate feeder–child interactions, to understand whether feeder interaction is maintaining inappropriate behaviours, and to determine if there is a behavioural element in the child's communications. Is the feeder obviously anxious, angry, frustrated? Is the child's feeding behaviour attracting attention? If so, the feeder will need to remain calm and remove incidents which are behavioural. This can be done by reducing obvious emotions, reactions, remaining silent or, where appropriate, leaving the room until the incident is over. See 'Behaviour and Communication' guidelines (pages 24–27).

9 ⋯ Help the feeder to read and **learn the child's communication signals** and reactions. This will help in understanding the child's likes and dislikes, whether the child is full or wants more, and anticipating problems. It will also help the child become an active communicator. Use the 'Stress Behaviours' checklist (page 20) or the 'Communication Behaviours' checklist (page 22) for detailed analysis.

10 ⋯ As much as possible, **give written guidelines**. This will facilitate the feeder's understanding and memory of techniques and recommendations.

Overview

A child needs to produce on average 300 sucks to obtain 2 ounces/60 millilitres of fluid. This represents a considerable amount of energy for normally developing children. For those with problems of reduced endurance, the amount of effort required to feed orally is considerable.

Causes and Contributory Factors

The main reasons for reduced endurance are cardiac problems, respiratory compromise and preterm birth.

Characteristics

Feeding sessions with children with reduced endurance tend to be either lengthy because of problems with co-ordinating the suck – swallow – breathe pattern, resulting in long, frequent pauses in sucking, or short, where the child 'turns off' because of the effort involved or as a coping mechanism. Some children will finish feeding early because their hunger has been momentarily satiated.

Changes in heart rate are easily evident if the child is on a monitor. The normal heart rate for infants is 100–160 beats per minute. Deviations are noted in, for example, bradycardia (slow heart rate), which in infants is considered to be below 100 beats per minute, and tachycardia (rapid heart rate), which in infants is estimated to be above 180 beats per minute.

Normal Development

It is important to remember that sleepiness in a young infant can be due to gestational age. Children do not generally demonstrate spontaneous alerting until gestational age of about 37 weeks.

While it can be difficult to estimate a child's heart rate if the child is not on a monitor, there are clinical indications which point to endurance problems. These include those listed in the following checklist. For example, colour changes in a child to red (not pink) or pale, which can be observed in the skin, lips, eyelids, hands and nails, indicate endurance problems. Use of the checklist will help in highlighting the presence of reduced endurance, but it is not exhaustive and the clinician will need to consider the individual history of the child when observing for indications of reduced endurance. A child need not demonstrate all signs to present with this problem. The checklist will also help the clinician and feeder to be aware of the child's signals and to anticipate problems. They should use the 'Stress Behaviours' checklist (page 20) for a more comprehensive analysis of the child's state, motor signals and autonomic signals.

97

CLINICAL INDICATIONS OF REDUCED ENDURANCE CHECKLIST

Part 1: *Medical Conditions and History*

AREA	NOTES
Current medical conditions and diagnoses	
1 ···History of attempts at oral feeding	
2 ···Success of attempts at oral feeding	
3 ···Reasons for abandonment of oral feeding, if relevant	

Part 2: *Clinical Observations*

FEATURES	PRESENT	ABSENT
Long feeding sessions		
Frequent, lengthy pauses in sucking		
Short feeding sessions		
Child 'shuts down', becomes drowsy		
Breathing shallow or chest recessed		
Colour changes to red or white		
Flaring nostrils		
Bradycardia or tachycardia		

Part 3: *Summary Analysis*

QUESTION	YES	NO
Are endurance problems present?		
Are endurance problems significant enough to affect the success of oral feeding?		
Is oral feeding currently contraindicated?		

Therapy guidelines

1 ⋯ Where oral feeding is contraindicated, **continue with tube feeding and normalization of sensation** where appropriate. Work on orofacial hypersensitivity/desensitization (see 'Orofacial Hypersensitivity' guidelines on pages 74–77). Work on tone, either increasing tone where hypotonia is present, or reducing tone where hypertonia is present. See 'Orofacial Hypotonia' guidelines on pages 79–81. Consult the paediatric occupational therapist and the paediatric physiotherapist so that overall body tone and motor skills can be addressed.

Touching and movement should be used generally and therapeutically to stimulate normal patterns of interaction, to decrease hypersensitivity, to reduce or increase tone and to normalize tube feeding when this takes place.

Most of these activities can be used even when a child is in the hospital and on a ventilator.

2 ⋯ Use of a consistent feeder is advisable so that the child's communications are consistently understood and responded to. When feeding orally, **always monitor the child's signals**, both non-intentional and intentional. Working with the child's system rather than against it will facilitate the oral feeding process. This helps the feeder and clinician to understand how the child is coping with oral feeding, and to anticipate problems. It also facilitates the child's awareness of himself as a communicator and promotes active communication.

3 ⋯ **Reduce environmental stimuli** to help with the child's internal organization concentration on feeding. Remove auditory stimuli by turning off the television, radio and so on; remove combined stimuli such as the presence of extra people in the room. Visual stimuli, such as a bright room, can function to alert the child, but with some younger infants, feeding at night or in the dark will help with internal organization.

4 ⋯ Where appropriate, **alert the child**. Use a well-lit room. Provide movement in any direction, such as just picking a baby up, gentle rocking from side to side, or gentle bouncing up and down. Unpredictable rhythms may encourage alertness. Use noise such as lively music, or voice with variations in pitch and degrees of animation.

Move the child into an upright position. Use touch, particularly light touch, and touch and movement combined. Wolf and Glass (1992) recommend activities such as tickling and stroking the child's palms, soles or head.

See 'Child Preparation' guidelines (pages 92–94).

99

5 ··· **Provide correct positioning** which will provide stability and support to make the feeding process less of an effort. An upright position can alert the child. A sidelying or curled position will provide a better covering of the epiglottis and conserve energy, which is particularly beneficial in cases of hypotonia such as Down's syndrome.

In a child with neck hyperextension, evaluate how much the child needs this hyperextension to maintain and protect the airway.

Bringing the head and body into greater flexion facilitates a number of oro-motor patterns such as sucking, lip seal and swallowing by aiding laryngeal closure. It also therefore helps to protect the airway.

6 ··· **Conserve the child's energy,** thereby promoting endurance and control. Do not play with the child before or after feeding. Do not dress the child before or after feeding. Do not bathe the child before or after feeding.

7 ··· **Do not try to increase the amount of oral intake** until the child is able to cope with very gradual changes. Oral feeding can be supplemented by following the oral feed experience with a tube feed if the child's system is able to cope. Alternatively, the oral feed can be topped up with tube feeds at night. Overnight tube feeds have a negative side, however, in that they do not serve to build up the child's association of the mouth with the stomach. The clinician must decide which system best meets the child's current and future needs.

8 ··· **Alter the feeding schedule.** Try shorter (reduced intake) but more frequent feeds, working from the point the child is able to cope with: if the child is only able to feed for five minutes, start at this point and increase the number of feeds, leaving time (about two hours) in between for the child to reorganize and re-energize (Wolf and Glass, 1992).

Allow the child to take half the amount and then provide a rest (no stimulation), continuing with the feed after 10 to 15 minutes.

Move to a demand schedule (feeding the child when he is hungry), which may lead to more vigorous feeding.

When altering the feeding schedule, monitor intake to ensure that nutritional requirements are met. Consult the paediatric dietician.

9 ··· **Use a soft teat,** as the child may tire quickly on a hard teat (Winstock, 1994; Wolf and Glass, 1992). However, the softer teat may not provide enough stimulation for the suck with some children, so try a number of teats where necessary.

10 ·· Where the child has no significant co-ordination or swallowing problems, and is not respiratorily compromised, **increase the flow of liquid** by enlarging the teat hole or using a fast-flow teat.

11 ·· In cases of reduced endurance particular problems centre around meeting the child's nutritional requirements. Where appropriate (usually with the older child), **provide nutritional supplements**, so that less effort is required for feeding. See 'Increasing Nutritional Intake' guidelines (pages 72–73). Refer to a paediatric dietician.

12 ·· Where children are breast-fed, and despite the advantages of breast-feeding (bonding, encouraging brain development, reducing incidence of necrotizing enterocolitis, providing antibodies), **discuss possible use of bottle feeding**, as this technique requires far less energy expenditure. The breast can continue to be used for comfort and bonding if the mother wishes.

13 ·· **Always monitor for signs of respiratory compromise and aspiration,** as these can be a particular problem in cases of reduced endurance. See 'Clinical Indications of Aspiration' checklist (page 15) and 'Clinical Indications of Respiratory Compromise' checklist (pages 112–113).

14 ·· Encourage the parents to have **realistic expectations**. If necessary, help carers to focus on other areas of change.

Gastro-oesophageal reflux overview

The mechanism of gastro-oesophageal reflux (GOR) is not clearly understood, but the term is used to define the return of the stomach contents from the oesophagus or stomach upwards. It can be mild, moderate, severe or profound and can cause a child to reject feeding as it makes the experience unpleasant.

Causes and Contributory Factors

Children who are prone to reflux include the following: children with increased muscle tone in the abdominal area (as with some types of cerebral palsy); premature babies (Neal, 1995, reports that gastrointestinal motility and gastric emptying are less well-developed in these children, which can contribute to reflux, among other conditions); and children with low tone of internal organs such as those presenting with Down's syndrome. Children who are either currently tube-fed or have a history of tube feeding may also be at risk. The naso- or orogastric tube to the stomach splits open the sphincter at the entrance to the stomach, increasing the likelihood of reflux.

Determining whether reflux is present is not solely dependent on the use of radiological techniques or medical investigations. Indeed, there are many occasions when reflux is actually present but this is not shown by videofluoroscopy or barium swallow procedures. This may be for a number of reasons:

▼ the child does not co-operate on the day of the investigation;
▼ the time limit may not be sufficient (reflux may not occur immediately);
▼ the bolus volume may not be large enough for reflux to be evident (the amount given does not reflect normal volumes of food the child receives);
▼ the reflux may not occur consistently;
▼ reflux may not occur on that particular occasion;
▼ the reflux may be mild in nature.

The clinician can observe clinical indications of reflux during the feeding process. These are outlined in the checklist in this section. Not all clinical indications need to be present for reflux to be occurring. It is also important, when using the checklist, to consider other conditions or limiting patterns which may be causing the clinical signs.

The clinician can also grade reflux, although this can be a difficult exercise: the child may not show obvious signs of reflux, and determining what constitutes significant reflux may pose problems. Grading of reflux should be based on the impact of reflux on the child and on feeding. This system is also useful in determining the success of therapeutic procedures and medical management. For a grading system to be useful, the clinician applying it to the individual child should be consistent and, where teams are involved, they should agree on the classifications used. The grading given below offers guidelines for this purpose, based on the following categorizations: clinical signs, frequency of occurrence, impact on the feeding process, impact on nutritional intake, results of radiological investigation and the child's attitude to feeding.

GRADING	
Normal **Grade 0 reflux**	• *No reflux present* • *No clinical signs evident* • *No reflux evident on radiological investigation*
Mild **Grade 1 reflux**	• *One or two clinical signs evident* • *Occurs infrequently* • *Does not affect feeding process* • *Nutritional intake not affected* • *No or insignificant reflux evident on radiological investigation* • *The child is not affected and continues with feeding*
Moderate **Grade 2 reflux**	• *More than two clinical signs evident in a number of areas* • *Occurs relatively infrequently* • *Nutritional intake not significantly affected* • *Child needs time to recover but feeding can continue* • *Reflux observed on radiological investigation, but not consistently* • *The child shows some reaction and resistance to feeding*
Severe **Grade 3 reflux**	• *Multiple clinical signs observed* • *Occurs frequently* • *Nutritional intake significantly affected* • *Significantly disrupts the feeding process and its effectiveness in terms of length of feeding and time for child's recovery* • *Easily and frequently evident on radiological investigation* • *The child demonstrates frequent aversive responses and resistance to feeding*
Profound **Grade 4 reflux**	• *Multiple clinical signs evident* • *Occurs continually* • *Nutrition significantly compromised* • *Feeding process significantly disrupted, with oral feeding contraindicated* • *Easily and consistently evident on radiological investigations* • *The child demonstrates continual aversive behaviour and refuses oral feeding*

CLINICAL INDICATIONS OF REFLUX CHECKLIST

NAME		DATE

Part 1: *Clinical Observations*

FEATURES	PRESENT	ABSENT
PHYSICAL • Extension/arching pattern • Flapping arms • Occurrence of strong flexor spasms which may precipitate or exacerbate episodes of reflux • Grimacing		
BEHAVIOURAL • Panic reaction when food enters oral cavity • Conflict: the child wants food, but also wants to avoid it because of a history of unpleasant experiences associated with feeding • Hypersensitivity to food. The child may not like getting food on hands and face, and therefore play with food is decreased • The child may control the feeding environment, eg. holding the spoon • Apparent discomfort following feeding which may persist for lengthy periods		
NUTRITIONAL • Decreased intake and/or reduced appetite. In particular, a reluctance to eat after taking only a small amount • Allowance of only a limited range of textures • Change in behaviour when intake is increased		
LARYNGEAL • Coughing/choking • Persistent phlegminess • Hoarse voice		
ASSOCIATED CONDITIONS • The presence of aspiration • Vomiting (not an essential sign)		

THE MANUAL OF PAEDIATRIC FEEDING PRACTICE

Part 2: *Medical Management and Investigation*

QUESTION	ANSWER
DRUGS • Is the child on any medications for reflux? If so, what are they? How has the child responded to their use?	
RADIOLOGY • Has radiological investigation been carried out? Which procedures? • With what results?	
OTHER INVESTIGATIONS • Have other procedures been attempted? Which ones, and with what results?	

Part 3: *Summary Observations*

QUESTION	ANSWER
Is gastro-oesophageal reflux likely to be present?	
Is it affecting oral feeding?	
Is it mild, moderate, severe or profound?	
Is oral feeding currently contraindicated?	

Therapy guidelines

1 ⋯ **Refer for videofluoroscopy and barium swallow,** which will help determine the absence or presence of reflux and aspiration, and the extent of these, in addition to identifying or discounting anatomical abnormalities and limiting patterns. It is becoming increasingly common for nasogastric tube-fed children to have a barium swallow procedure conducted via the tube. The clinician must be aware that the findings from this procedure when the tube is used cannot be regarded as a blanket finding. The tube to the stomach splits the sphincter open, which increases the likelihood of reflux. When children move on to oral feeding, if reflux is suspected, the procedure should be repeated via the oral route. See 'Videofluoroscopy' guidelines (pages 166–167).

2 ⋯ **Refer for medical assessment and management.** Investigations may include monitoring of PH levels (acidity or alkalinity of body secretions), search for allergies and clinical trials of drugs either singly or in combination. The child may in some cases be referred for surgical management such as nissen fundiplication (where the stomach sphincter is wrapped so that the child cannot vomit). This procedure, while common with children who have had a gastrostomy, is not always effective in eliminating or reducing reflux.

3 ⋯ **Provide improved positioning.** With some children, improved positioning can make a great deal of difference to controlling and/or decreasing the effects of reflux, thanks to increased internal and external stability and the effects of gravity which aid digestion and reduce the potential for, or effects of, reflux.

The general rule is that the more upright and flexed (including chin tuck) the child is, the less potential there is for reflux. Individual children may respond differently to changes in positions, so try several. Positioning should also be upright and flexed for about half an hour after meals, and as much as possible at mealtimes. Reflux and aspiration can occur long after feeding.

While the stomach should not be compressed, Evans-Morris and Dunn-Klein (1987) recommend a very forward (flexed) position (30 to 45 degrees) after meals, using a wedge or standing frame. They feel the pressure on the stomach can in fact aid digestion and chest expansion for fuller breathing. Similarly, Wolf and Glass (1992) recommend anywhere from a 30 to a 90 degree flexed position after meals. It is best to try out different post-feed positions with the individual child and evaluate which suits him best. Consult the child's paediatric occupational therapist about seating and positioning.

4 ··· **Reduce tone and tension in the abdominal area,** if appropriate. Unco-ordination of the diaphragm or spasms in the abdominal area can precipitate or contribute to reflux. Work on developing respiratory and phonatory control. Consult the child's paediatric physiotherapist for specific advice.

5 ··· **Reduce environmental stimuli** so that the child can concentrate and relax during feeding. Such stimuli include auditory stimuli, such as televisions and radios, visual stimuli, such as bright lights, and combined stimuli such as the presence of extra people. Stimuli can gradually be reintroduced as the child's coping skills improve.

6 ··· As reflux may be triggered or contributed to by hypersensitivity or desensitization, particularly where there is a history of tube feeding and where there has been reduced oral feeding, **focus on normalizing sensation**. This is particularly important where the child has limited or non-existent experience of oral feeding. Help the child develop mouthing skills by facilitating him in exploring his hands, rubber toys and so on. See 'Orofacial Hypersensitivity/Desensitization' guidelines (pages 74–77).

7 ··· **Thicken the feed** to reduce the possibility of reflux. Thin liquids tend to be more difficult for children with unstable neurological states and limiting oro-motor patterns. Thicker feeds provide greater sensory input and move more slowly, therefore providing the child with greater control of the bolus. The increased weight of the food should also help keep it in the stomach and out of the oesophagus. Evans-Morris and Dunn-Klein (1987) point out that thickening feeds may in fact increase the chances of reflux, as the food stays longer in the stomach. However, it appears that children who have their feed thickened are generally more comfortable. Add a tablespoon of dry rice to two ounces (60 millilitres) of formula and enlarge the teat if the child is bottle-fed (Alexander, 1987; Winstock, 1994); use commercial thickeners; reduce the liquid content when making food by adding less liquid or cooking off to thicken; add natural thickeners such as apple sauce to liquid.

8 ··· If a child has reduced or non-existent oral intake, start by offering small amounts of food. With oral feeders, **reduce the amount fed**, as the child may tolerate more easily small amounts of food in the stomach at a time. Supplement through the tube or by increasing the frequency of meals.

9 ··· **Reduce the bolus size** offered to the child for the same reason as in (8). Try increasing the size as the child's coping skills develop.

107

▼

10 ·· **Explore the child's communication signals** to investigate whether reflux and vomiting are being used on a behavioural level. See the 'Communication Behaviours' checklist (page 22).

11 ·· The **use of distracters** during feeding may help to take the child's mind off reflux.

12 ·· **Use food play**, where the child can experience food and utensils without pressure and with more control. Try messy play with food, where appropriate. Use a non-slip plastic mat or a plastic bath. With the child who does not like being dirty, start with less sloppy food. Use 'pretend' and imaginary play such as feeding the doll, teddy or the feeder.

13 ·· **Encourage positive imaging and a relaxed attitude to food.** Read happy stories which involve food as the theme. Tell of happy events involving food, such as picnics or trips to the beach (Evans-Morris and Dunn-Klein, 1987). Encourage the feeder to relax at feeding time and to imagine the feeding process, the child and the feeder positively.

14 ·· Where allergies are suspected, refer for dietetic and medical assessment. Evans-Morris and Dunn-Klein (1987) suggest **exploring the response to different formulas**. This should only be done under dietetic and medical advice. They recommend testing each type of formula on a weekly basis and monitoring the child's positive or negative responses on a variety of levels. Try out meat-based, soya and milk-based feeds and so on. Children who are prone to allergic reactions may include, according to Evans-Morris and Dunn-Klein *(ibid)* those with a family history of allergies, frequent colds and other congestion, increased mucus production in the airway and digestive system, dark circles under the eyes, chronic middle ear infections and inconsistencies in physical, emotional or behavioural characteristics.

Nasal reflux overview

Reflux through the nasal passages occurs when the food, rather than entering the pharynx and oesophagus, travels up into the nasal cavity.

Causes and Contributory Factors

Wolf and Glass (1992) report that nasal reflux can be contributed to by a number of factors, including gravity, increased tone and hyperextension, cleft hard and soft palates, short or poorly elevated velopharynx (soft palate) and problems with co-ordinating the suck–swallow–breathe pattern.

Therapy guidelines

1 ··· **Assess the hard and soft palate.** Elevation of the soft palate is an important area to evaluate as it functions to seal off the nasal cavity. Conduct a direct orofacial assessment, looking at both the structure and function of the hard and soft palates. Check for the presence of cleft. Assess elevation of the soft palate. Listen to the child's speech, vocalizations and crying to check for a nasal imbalance.

2 ··· **Concentrate on the main problem area.** This could be co-ordination of the suck–swallow–breathe sequence, hypertonia or presence of a cleft. See 'Co-ordination of Sucking, Swallowing, Breathing', 'Orofacial Hypertonia', 'Cleft Palate' guidelines as appropriate.

3 ··· Where the velopharynx is short or poorly elevated, **focus on soft palate function**. Provide sensory input and stimulation. Starting at the juncture between the hard and soft palates, gradually move further back on to the soft palate; this should help the palate elevate. Use a finger, wet cotton swab or toothbrush to stimulate the area. Cold stimuli such as an ice stick (frozen water in a plastic straw with the plastic then removed to reveal an inch of stick) applied to this area will also help.

With an older child, a palatal prosthesis may help with closure and control. Consult a specialist therapist or clinic (Evans-Morris and Dunn-Klein, 1987).

Onward referral to ENT for pharyngeal flap surgery may be an option if the child is medically stable (Evans-Morris and Dunn-Klein, 1987).

4 ··· **Provide appropriate positioning.** Focus on upright positioning which will help with the correct descent of the bolus. Chin tuck should help reduce reflux. Correct positioning after as well as during feeds is important. See 'Gastro-oesophageal Reflux' guidelines (pages 106–108).

5 ··· **Thicken feeds** with cereal, mashed potato, cornflour and water, or commercial thickener, to help the child improve control of the bolus. See 'Gastro-oesophageal Reflux' guidelines (pages 106–108).

RESPIRATORY COMPROMISE

Overview

The importance of respiration to the feeding process cannot be underestimated, and the child's breathing can often be an indicator of potential problems in this area. Respiratory compromise means increased work for breathing, which usually results in poor co-ordination of the suck–swallow–breathe pattern and may contribute to a number of other conditions.

Normal Development

The normal respiratory rate for preterm babies is about 40 to 60 breaths per minute (bpm). It is also important to remember that in infants the space in the oral cavity and oropharynx is reduced. The space gradually develops through childhood. Young infants without respiration problems are usually good at feeding as they breathe through the nasal passages and use the oral cavity for feeding.

Causes and Contributory Factors

Respiratory compromise can be caused or contributed to by a number of reasons, including structural abnormalities such as tracheal stenosis and musculoskeletal abnormalities; an unstable neurological state typified by irregular or shallow breathing; respiratory disease, such as Infant Respiratory Distress Syndrome (IRDS) which is evident in very rapid breathing (tachypnoea) or Broncho-Pulmonary Dysplasia (BPD), commonly seen after prolonged ventilation of premature babies (the incidence of IRDS has fallen with the use of antenatal steroids: Neal, 1995). The volume of food in the stomach may impede respiration (Neal, 1995).

It is important to determine whether the child's respiratory status is conducive to oral feeding, and this decision needs to be made by taking into account medical conditions and management, and clinical observations. Where the child is on a monitor and supplementary oxygen, it is relatively easy to determine how well he is coping, both at rest and during exertion (for example, when feeding), by watching the monitors for changes. However, not all children with respiratory compromise will have this facility, so it is doubly important for the clinician to attend to clinical signs which may indicate how the child is coping on this level.

The following checklist is intended to provide the clinician with some guidelines. Not all children who are compromised in the manner indicated will exhibit all the signs listed. For example, a child's rate of breathing may be acceptable, but with a shallow or an irregular pattern. Wolf and Glass (1992) point out, however, that rate of breathing should be monitored where possible, during active feeding and during pauses in sucking.

The clinician should note that clinical signs may be caused or contributed to by a problem in another area, and this possibility should be taken into account when observing the individual child.

▼

CLINICAL INDICATIONS OF RESPIRATORY COMPROMISE CHECKLIST

NAME	DATE

Part 1: Medical Conditions and History

QUESTION	ANSWER
Note relevant medical history.	
What is medical and respiratory status?	
What is current medical management (including oxygen supplementation, monitoring)?	
Has oral feeding been attempted? If so, what was the result? Why was it stopped?	

Part 2: Clinical Observations

FACTOR	YES	NO
RESPIRATORY • Is irregular or shallow breathing evident? • Is a high respiration rate evident? If so, is this at rest? Only during feeding? • Is endurance reduced?		
NUTRITIONAL • Is weight gain compromised even if the child is successfully feeding orally (but using too much energy to feed)?		
ORAL STRUCTURES AND FUNCTIONS • Is the suck–swallow–breathe pattern unco-ordinated? • Does the child take frequent pauses while sucking? • Is the tongue sufficiently retracted to impinge on breathing?		
HEART RATE • Is heart rate rapid (tachycardia) or too slow (bradycardia)?		
ASSOCIATED CONDITIONS • Is aspiration present? If so, to what extent?		

Part 3: *Summary Observations*

QUESTION	ANSWER
Does medical history support the introduction/continuation of oral feeding?	
Do clinical observations support the introduction/continuation of oral feeding?	
Should oral feeding commence/continue?	

Therapy guidelines

1 ⋯ **Oral feeding may be contraindicated.** In inappropriate conditions, aspiration, apnoea and bradycardia may occur and therefore postponement, either temporarily or permanently, of oral feeding aims may be advisable. Such conditions include those where the child is autonomically unstable, the child's respiratory status does not support oral feeding, or where the child feeds orally but uses too much energy in doing so, thus compromising weight gain. In these situations it is important (1) to maintain a focus on tube feeding: long-term tube feeders should be considered and recommended for a gastrostomy; (2) to focus on reducing tone and hypersensitivity, where appropriate; (3) to consider the use of supplements (consult the child's paediatric dietician); and (4) to encourage realistic feeder expectations.

2 ⋯ **Focus on specific problem areas.** For example, highlight the co-ordination of the suck–swallow–breathe pattern, aspiration or tongue retraction, where appropriate. As respiratory problems often result in endurance problems, see 'Reduced Endurance' guidelines (pages 99–101).

3 ⋯ Where oral feeding may be potentially unsafe until respiratory issues are resolved, **provide non-nutritional therapeutic activities** where possible. Use small amounts of fluid and a syringe and slowly release into the oral cavity tiny amounts of fluid (measured in tenths of a millilitre). Where nutritive sucking is decreased, develop non-nutritive sucking. Use a.dummy, a teat blocked with wet gauze (to prevent air entering) or a finger. Grade changes with these children especially carefully.

4 ⋯ When working with children with respiratory compromise, **always monitor autonomic, motor and state reactions and behaviours** extremely carefully. Respiratory rate (while awake) should not be above 70 to 75 bpm before beginning feeding and, if it reaches 80 to 85 bpm during feeding, feeding should be stopped (Brodsky, 1993). Where it remains elevated, finish feeding. Where it falls, continue cautiously. See the 'Stress Behaviours' checklist for detailed monitoring (page 20).

5 ⋯ Some children have problems with co-ordinating the suck–swallow–breathe pattern because of respiratory difficulties, and this can often lead to feeding-induced apnoea. The tendency is for prolonged sucking or bursts of short sucking to occur. **Introduce external pacing**, where the feeder breaks the suction and defines the rhythm. Impose a break after two or three sucks by removing the teat, leaving the teat in place but inserting a finger into the mouth to break the suction, or tilting the bottle downwards to stop the flow of liquid

(Wolf and Glass, 1992). Pacing may only be essential during the latter part of feeding, when the child is having more difficulties co-ordinating.

If external pacing is not possible, remove the teat after the first sign of respiratory difficulty to help the child learn to co-ordinate the suck–swallow–breathe pattern for himself. The feeder should regularly test the child's self-pacing by leaving the bottle in the mouth longer than normal.

6 · · · **Provide correct positioning** to provide stability and make feeding less of an effort. With infants and small children, a sidelying or curled position will provide better covering of the epiglottis and require less energy expenditure. This is suitable for children with cardiac problems and low tone.

For children who arch or extend back, position them *en face* on the feeder's lap, with the feeder's legs supported by a chair. This will prevent the back arching but let the child have room to extend his arms and turn his head. This is good for children with hyperextension caused by lung disease such as BPD.

It is always important in children with neck hyperextension to evaluate how much hyperextension they need to maintain and protect the airway: the child may need some neck extension to breathe. See 'Positioning' guidelines (pages 82–83).

7 · · · **Experiment with breast-feeding** where this is developmentally appropriate. Children who are prone to ear infections may benefit from breast-feeding, which requires wider jaw excursions than bottle-feeding and can function to keep the eustachian tubes patent. However, this must be balanced against potential for reduced endurance, as breast-feeding requires more effort than bottle-feeding because of the necessity for wider jaw excursions.

8 · · · Where there is increased effort and energy expenditure, the child may benefit from the **provision of nutritional supplements**, particularly if intake is not increased or sufficient with the oral method of feeding. See 'Increasing Nutritional Intake' guidelines (pages 72–73). Refer to a paediatric dietician.

9 · · · Wolf and Glass (1992) recommend considering **the provision of additional respiratory support** by using supplemental oxygen continuously or solely during feeding, done under guidance of the appropriate professional. Assess the child's response, before, during and after feeding, to the use of supplemental oxygen to determine its benefits. Consult the appropriate medical and nursing specialities.

Overview

Excessive drooling is messy and socially unacceptable. It may occur in particular following meals or during activities which require concentration, and with some children may be continuous. Drooling tends to be regarded as an infantile behaviour and, as Ray et al (1983) point out, there is therefore the potential for underestimating a child's ability because of drooling.

Disadvantages of Reduced Saliva Control

Reduced maintenance of saliva in the mouth can have a significant negative impact. As saliva assists with tasting (Winstock, 1994), the child's ability to taste will be reduced. Oral hygiene (bad breath, gum and dental problems) can be a problem (Ray *et al*, 1983; Winstock, 1994). Feeding and oro-motor efficiency can be reduced as saliva helps ready the bolus for chewing and swallowing, regulates acidity in the gut and initiates the digestion of carbohydrates (Winstock, 1994). Dehydration can result from excessive fluid loss (Ray *et al*, 1983; Winstock, 1994). Speech problems can develop because of the reduced oro–motor control, and clarity can be affected as saliva functions to lubricate the tongue and lips during speech. Physical appearance can be affected and social interaction with the child by peers and adults may be reduced or otherwise negatively affected when a child drools a lot (Strawbridge-Domaracki and Sisson, 1990). The child may suffer from negative feelings such as embarrassment, frustration and decreased self-confidence. Materials that the child comes into contact with may have repeatedly to be cleaned, washed or replaced when excessive drooling occurs.

Normal Development

Alexander (1987), Arvedson (1993b) and Brodsky (1993) give the following guidelines on the normal development of swallowing as outlined below. Infants produce very little saliva until age three months and by six to nine months they can usually control it relatively well, with the exception of activities that require concentration, and when cutting teeth. Improved saliva control develops along with improved oro–motor stability and muscle control. By age 15 months, drooling usually only occurs with some fine motor tasks. Spillage continues with food until age 24 months. There continues to be minor spillage up to three years of age, but in general saliva is well-controlled within the oral cavity.

Causes and Contributory Factors

Contrary to popular belief, children with difficulties in controlling saliva do not suffer from overproduction of saliva, but with transporting and in general controlling it within the oral cavity. There may be a number of reasons for drooling. Reduced saliva control can indicate a swallowing dysfunction. Ekedahl *et al* (1978) demonstrate that neurologically impaired droolers have abnormalities in swallowing, usually at the first stage, which is where the saliva is transported to the back of the mouth consciously and voluntarily. Limiting oro-motor patterns such as reduced mouth closure or poor tongue-tip elevation (to help initiate the swallow) can affect the child's control. Abnormal tone as in hypertonia (which restricts oro-motor movement) and hypotonia (which prevents sustained and controlled movement), can interfere with swallowing (Ray *et al*, 1983) and oro-motor sensation and feedback. Reduced physical stability, particularly with regard to head and neck control and jaw stability, can affect the child's ability to co-ordinate and control oro-motor structures and functions. Finally, children who are developmentally delayed may have a tendency to drool (Ray *et al*, 1983).

Treatment

There are three main methods of treating a child with reduced saliva control: behaviour modification, oro-motor therapy and surgery. Each has proved relatively successful, but no approach has eliminated drooling in children with severe saliva control problems. Ray *et al* (1983) have pointed out that older children may require longer periods of intervention when treating drooling.

Brodsky (1993) provides a quantification of drooling based on frequency of occurrence and area affected. This quantification has been adapted and developed below to help with determining the severity of drooling and the effects of therapeutic and medical management. The contributory categorizations are frequency, area affected, parental perceptions, child awareness and oral dysfunction. Use of this grading system needs to take into account the normal development of saliva control, as outlined above. What is normal or expected for a four-year-old is far different from what is common and expected of a 12-month-old.

A grading system is only useful when its application is consistent for individual children. When working in teams, it is beneficial for agreement on what constitutes the separate levels to be achieved. Not all criteria need to be met for a child's saliva control problem to be assigned to a specific level.

GRADING	
Normal **Grade 0 control**	• *Normal control – never drools* • *Within developmental level*
Mild **Grade 1 control**	• *Drools on to lip only* • *Drools on occasion, not daily* • *Parent not concerned* • *Child not aware or unconcerned* • *No oro-motor problems observed*
Moderate **Grade 2 control**	• *Drools on to lip and chin* • *Everyday occurrence with some dry episodes* • *Parent comments on drooling but not significantly concerned; makes some attempts to control* • *Child may be aware but makes no or few comments or displays little concern about drooling* • *May have oro-motor problems but not significantly affecting control*
Severe **Grade 3 control**	• *Clothing is soiled* • *Drooling is continuous* • *Parent concerned and frequently wiping or requesting child to control drooling* • *Child aware and makes frequent attempts to clean or requests cleaning* • *Oro-motor problems evident and contributing to drooling*
Profound **Grade 4 control**	• *Drools on to hands and equipment such as toys and table* • *Drooling is continuous* • *Parent very concerned and constantly wiping or asking child to control* • *Child anxious, with effects on concentration or socialization. Makes constant effort or requests for cleaning* • *Oro-motor problems evident and significant in their impact on drooling*

Therapy guidelines

1 ··· With mild cases, **no treatment** is the suitable option.

2 ··· Where there is a problem, **focus on reducing an open mouth posture**, where appropriate. Ensure nasal breathing is not compromised and that the child does not require an open mouth posture to maintain an airway. With older and cognitively able children, reminding them verbally to close their mouths can help and this approach also encourages the child to take responsibility for saliva control. This approach should be used in combination with a reinforcement/reward system.

Provide examples of a closed mouth using mirrors, mouth puppets and so on. Provide experience and practice of a closed mouth by using external support (a finger under the lips and so on). Help develop increased closure and approximation through use of increasingly small food items which can be sucked. Start with frozen lollipops or juice sticks and move on to liquorice sticks, then spaghetti and so on. Ensure that the child can cope orally with these items.

With spoon feeding, allow time for lip activity. The spoon should not be removed rapidly or scraped against the gum ridge.

Develop lip and cheek motor skills through blowing games (with bubbles, candles and so on) and use of straws.

See 'Lip Seal' guidelines (pages 61–63) and 'Cheek Stability' guidelines (pages 28–29) for further details.

3 ··· **Focus on the primary problem area:** for example, poor lip seal, head and neck control, tonal abnormalities, jaw stability or a swallowing dysfunction, which may be causing or significantly contributing to reduced saliva control. See 'Lip Seal', 'Orofacial Hypotonia', 'Jaw Instability', or 'Co-ordination of Sucking, Swallowing and Breathing' guidelines as relevant.

4 ··· **Provide sensory input** to the cheek, lip and jaw areas to increase sensation and thereby facilitate saliva control. This is especially important in conditions of hypotonia. Apply firm but gentle pressure in circular movements around the mouth; use a toothbrush (either child's or trainer) to increase sensation; use a cap with chin strap, as outlined below. See 'Orofacial Hypertonia' (pages 78–79) or 'Orofacial Hypotonia' guidelines (pages 79–81), as relevant.

5 ··· **Focus on the development of jaw stability.** As both head control and jaw stability improve, so will the child's control over saliva. When this technique is effective, automatic control over drooling should develop. Ensure good positioning. Evans-Morris and Dunn-Klein (1987) recommend the use of a cap with a chin strap to help provide jaw stability through mild resistance (the strap should not keep the jaw closed when in place). Reduce the tension on the strap as jaw stability and saliva control improve. See 'Jaw Instability' guidelines (pages 57–58) for specific details.

6 ··· **Ensure appropriate positioning** which is essential for increased head control and therefore control of saliva. Provide frequent and continuing experience of an upright position. Short, frequent periods of such positioning during relaxing time (eg. watching a video) without pressure to swallow will help the child to experience normal saliva control (Winstock, 1994).

7 ··· **Stimulate and assist a swallow** directly to help the child with control.

▼ **Tap the tip of the tongue and the spot on the hard palate that the tip of the tongue touches (Evans-Morris and Dunn-Klein, 1987). Repeat if necessary.**

▼ **Firmly but gently, stroke a finger down the child's throat following the floor of the mouth.**

▼ **Remind the child verbally to swallow where the child is capable of controlling and organizing this.**

8 ··· If appropriate, **develop improved chewing patterns** which will help with oro-motor control. See 'Chewing' guidelines (pages 30–32).

9 ··· **Reduce the use of citrus and sweet foods** which tend to increase saliva production.

10 ·· When a child's mouth is wet it may be essential to clean and dry it if the child is not able to do this for himself. Because the way in which it is done may make all the difference where progress is concerned, Winstock (1994) recommends clear **wiping** practice:

▼ **Do not push the child's head back when wiping – maintain a good trunk and head position.**

▼ **Do not wipe excessively, but only when necessary.**

▼ **Do not approach the child quickly and wipe suddenly and without warning. Give a verbal, visual and/or tactile cue.**

▼ **Do not use a large cloth, as this will stimulate further saliva production. Use a small tight wad of absorbent material.**

▼ **Do not use light movements, as they are overstimulating. Wipe the side affected with three firm dabs.**

▼ **Do not wipe the whole oral or facial area. Concentrate on the affected area.**

▼ **Do not tell the child to swallow – this may be difficult and may make the child anxious. Verbal reminding should only be used when the child is capable of swallowing by himself, is aware of and affected by his drooling, and will respond to such techniques without this negatively affecting his confidence.**

11 ·· **Increase the child's awareness.**

▼ **Teach the concepts of wet and dry, and open and closed, where this is developmentally appropriate (Evans-Morris and Dunn-Klein, 1987), using everyday activities such as washing up, opening doors, relevant storybooks and so on.**

▼ **Focus on dry times when concentrating on the child, increase the child's awareness of these and praise him for them.**

▼ **Do a favoured activity such as reading or playing a turn-taking game. Stop when the child dribbles and restart when it is under control.**

12 ·· If possible, **let the child take responsibility** for the dribbling by monitoring himself and wiping his own mouth. If the child does not like carrying wads of material, sweatbands may be more acceptable.

13 ·· Behaviour modification programmes can help if a child can swallow saliva and is motivated to do so. **Use reward systems** to reinforce mouth closure. Time the child from when he closes his mouth and help him to extend the time he can do so.

14 ·· With older children, other options include **medication and surgery**. Procedures used include excision or ligation of the parotid and submandibular glands, and division of the parasympathic fibres (Goode and Smith, 1970). Surgical techniques have had varying success in reducing drooling. Behaviour modification techniques and oro-motor therapy should always be attempted before considering surgical intervention. Consult the paediatrician or ENT specialist.

15 ·· Several **training devices** are available but may only have short-term effects. Further information can be obtained from a specialized clinic or speech and language therapist.

16 ·· **Specialized clothing** is available, if necessary (see Winstock, 1994, page 104).

17 ·· **Have realistic expectations.** With some children with reduced control, it may be unrealistic to expect saliva control during activities which require concentration; drooling may be a result of the need to maintain an oral airway.

121

Overview

Normal Development: Oro-motor Skills

The developmental guidelines outlined below are based on observations by Alexander (1987), Evans-Morris and Dunn-Klein (1987) and Winstock (1994). Removal of food from a spoon begins with the introduction of puréed foods and, until age six to nine months, is achieved by sucking, the lips not assisting with actual removal. When food is pushed out by the child, this is usually because the in–out suckle pattern is predominating, in combination with the relative inactivity of the lips. Around age seven to eight months, the lips begin to take a more active part in posturing for the spoon, providing stability and assisting with removal. Initially, the lower lip elevates and protrudes.

This is followed by lowering and protrusion of the upper lip. At this age, the child will also recognize the spoon by touch or sight, and the jaw will become stable, the mouth open and the tongue still in preparation for the loaded spoon. The sucking pattern continues to predominate, but other structures are now playing a larger part in the process. At age 10 months, the upper and lower lips draw inwards as the spoon is removed. By 12 months, general development in tone, muscle strength and stability makes for more advanced and co-ordinated sequences of movement. At 15 months, the teeth begin to play a greater part in spoon-feeding when the upper incisors are used to clean the lower lip as it draws inward. From age 24 months, the tongue is used to clean food from the labial area; tongue movement is now independent of jaw stability.

Normal Development: Self-help Skills

The following guidelines for self-feeding are based on Evans-Morris and Dunn-Klein (1987) and Winstock (1994). Self-feeding by spoon should only be taught after finger-feeding occurs at around age six to nine months, when the child will pick up food. Arvedson and Christensen (1993), however, recommend that it can be introduced from age four to six months. At age nine to 12 months, the child plays with food and can hold a spoon. From 12 to 18 months, the child can bring the spoon to the mouth, but full control is not yet achieved and the child will tend to overturn the spoon, losing the food. From age 18 to 24 months, control develops and, though spillage continues, it is less significant. Spoon-feeding is usually independent by two years of age.

Causes and Contributory Factors

Problems with spoon-feeding and self-feeding arise predominantly from physical and tonal abnormalities, such as reduced head, neck and trunk stability; hypertonia and the tendency to hyperextend; hypotonia and reduced sensation and therefore reduced response to and control of the stimulus; and limiting oro-motor patterns.

Therapy guidelines

1 ··· Introduce spoon-feeding by **using familiar, but thickened liquids**. This may be messy, but the child will be more keen to try with familiar foods than with unfamiliar ones. Use foods and tastes the child is accustomed to; reduce the liquid content of foods by cooking or using less blending; thicken by adding baby cereal, cornflour and so on; add a small amount of a new taste to a familiar taste, for example, to yogurt.

2 ··· **Use an appropriate spoon.** The spoon should be shallow-bowled, as this will make it easier to remove food than with a deep spoon. A narrow spoon will mean less food entering the mouth, making for easier placement and giving the child greater control (leading to the development of chewing). A metal spoon will also mean easier removal of food than from a plastic one, but some children do not respond well to the coldness of a metal spoon. Winstock (1994) recommends piling food high on a spoon, which may make for easier removal, but be aware that this technique may restrict tongue movement in children with dysfunctional skills or limiting patterns.

3 ··· **Face the child and present the spoon at mouth level.** This will prepare the child for the food, and his ability to see it and receive it at the right level will mean that there will be fewer limiting patterns (such as extension) present to affect placement and control of the bolus (Winstock, 1994).

4 ··· **Do not remove food from the spoon by scraping it against the gum ridge or teeth.** This is a common practice with children who have dysfunctional feeding, generally and naturally used to speed up the process. However, it reduces the child's control and active participation in feeding, along with the child's opportunities to develop more refined oro-motor skills.

5 ··· **Facilitate and prompt the child's spoon-feeding himself.** Provide support at the shoulder, elbow or wrist. This support should be reduced gradually (from heavy to light, from full hand to one finger) as the child develops control. Consult the paediatric occupational therapist.

123

Checklist and Grading

Use the following checklist to evaluate the suck and its related characteristics. The swallow can be assessed in detail by referring to the checklist on page 140. When categorizing the suck, it is not essential for it to meet all the criteria in the relevant section. Determining the characteristics of the suck is important for determining its management.

The sucking function can also be graded into levels of difficulty based on a number of classifications: contribution to associated problems such as chest infections and aspiration; effect on the feeding process, specifically length, and disruption; effect on nutritional intake and weight gain; ability to handle food consistencies; presence and extent of oro-motor dysfunction(s), such as unco-ordination and tongue movement; laryngeal activity, such as coughing and choking; and the child's response to feeding.

When grading against these guidelines, it is important to remember that other factors, such as aspiration, reflux or respiratory compromise, may be affecting feeding. The clinician must take this into account when grading, and grade with reference to the sucking function only. To be useful, grading must be consistent when applied to an individual child (there must be a constant clinician applying the grading). Where teams are involved, the team members must agree on the classifications. Grading is only useful in these circumstances – and for evaluating the effect of therapeutic management.

GRADING	
Normal **Grade 0 suck**	• *No dysfunction evident*
Mild **Grade 1 suck**	• *No significant history of aspiration or chest infections* • *No significant impact on feeding, nutritional intake or child's attitude to feeding* • *Minimal oro-motor problems* • *Infrequent coughing*
Moderate **Grade 2 suck**	• *Occasional chest infections and indications of aspiration* • *Feeding process disrupted regularly but not to a significant degree, as child continues; feeding takes slightly longer than normal* • *Nutritional intake and weight gain below normal but extra supplements not required* • *Child evidences difficulties on swallow with thin liquids only* • *Oro-motor difficulties present and affecting suck* • *Child coughs or chokes on regular, but not consistent, basis* • *Child shows some negative responses to feeding*
Severe **Grade 3 suck**	• *Frequent chest infections, with bouts of pneumonia; aspiration clinically evident* • *Feeding process significantly disrupted and oral feeding difficult* • *Nutritional intake and weight gain significantly compromised; child requires supplements or tube feeding top-up* • *Significant oro-motor difficulties present, affecting suck* • *Coughing, choking and gagging consistent and frequent features of feeding* • *Child displays aversive reactions to oral feeding which affect the process*
Profound **Grade 4 suck**	• *Oral feeding contraindicated* • *Persistent chest infections, pneumonia and significant aspiration* • *Feeding process ineffective because of sucking dysfunction, in terms of effort expended for weight gained* • *Constant choking or gagging response to oral feed* • *Child refuses oral feed*

SUCK EVALUATION CHECKLIST

NAME		DATE

Part 1: *Clinical Observations*

FEATURES	PRESENT	ABSENT
THE SUCK • Is a non-nutritive suck present (use a finger or teat to check for this)? • Is a nutritive suck present? • Is the suck co-ordinated? • What is the ratio of sucks to breaths?		
ORO-MOTOR • Are limiting functions present which affect the suck? • Are oro-motor structures normal?		

Part 2: *Characteristics of the Suck*

QUESTION	ANSWER
• Is the suck normal or dysfunctional?	
CO-ORDINATION OF THE SUCK–SWALLOW–BREATHE PATTERN • Does the child pause for breaths irregularly? • Does the child need time to recover? • Is the suck–swallow–breathe sequence generally unrhythmical? • Does tone fluctuate? • Is respiratory status compromised? • Are limiting patterns such as tongue retraction present? Specify. • Is the child's neurological state depressed? • Is the child hypersensitive or desensitized orally? • Is aspiration present?	

126

QUESTION	ANSWER
SUCK INITIATION • Can the child inhibit the rooting (search for teat) reflex to begin sucking? • Is hypertonia present? • Is extreme mouth opening present? • Is the child unable to close the mouth to initiate the suck? • Is the tongue excessively protruded or elevated? • Is lip seal achieved? • Is the jaw stable?	
SUCKLING • Has the child reached appropriate milestones (around 6 months) for sucking to be developing? • Is tongue movement predominantly in–out rather than up–down? • Is sucking characterized by a short burst (3–5 sucks) followed by a swallow, rather than long (10–30) bursts? • Does the tongue protrude excessively?	
WEAK SUCK • Does the child tire easily during feeding? • Is nutritional intake compromised? • Does feeding start with a strong suck which gradually weakens over the course of feeding? • Is hypotonia present? • Is the child respiratorily compromised? • Are anatomical problems (eg. palatal clefts, micrognathia) present which would affect sucking efficiency?	

Co-ordination of the suck–swallow–breathe pattern overview

The human feeding sequence requires the co-ordination of over 20 different muscles for the transport of food to the stomach from the mouth (Dodds, 1989; Palmer, 1989). Problems with co-ordinating the suck–swallow–breathe pattern can dramatically affect the success of the feeding process and the child's attitude to it.

Causes and Contributory Factors

Difficulties in this area can be caused by tonal abnormalities, orofacial hypersensitivity and desensitization, limiting oral patterns, such as tongue retraction, respiratory diseases resulting in compromise, reduced endurance, unstable neurological states, progressive neurological problems (such as Rett's syndrome) and premature introduction of oral feeding.

Normal Development

The following outline is based on Alexander (1987) and Wolf and Glass (1992). The newborn child can breathe and swallow at the same time. Non-nutritive sucking is usually present at around 28 weeks' gestation and characterized by a single suck followed by a long pause. This gradually develops to nutritive sucking, which starts at around 35 weeks, with continuous sucking bursts of more than 30 seconds. This develops into a pattern of intermittent sucking bursts (one per second) punctuated by regular pauses. This gradually develops (to two sucks per second, three sucks per second and so on), followed by a regular pause to swallow and breathe. By age three months, the ratio of sucks to swallows/breaths has increased to more than 20 sucks, and by six months even longer sequences are evident. By age 12 months, developing stability and co-ordination provide a base for co-ordinated, refined and sequenced oro-motor activity.

Feeding Stages

Four distinct stages in the human feeding cycle have been identified. The following is an outline of Reilly *et al's* (1995) summary of these stages. The preparatory or anticipatory phase constitutes food-getting and anticipatory reactions. The oral stage involves bolus management and transfer, including sucking, chewing and so on. The pharyngeal phase incorporates swallowing. Finally, the oesophageal phase begins with the relaxation and opening of the upper oesophageal sphincter. Stages 1 and 2 are sometimes classified jointly as the oral–preparatory phase.

Therapy guidelines

[1] ··· Consult medical staff to **rule out medical problems** which may be causing or contributing to the problem.

[2] ··· **Check swallowing function.** See 'Swallowing Function' Checklist (page 140).

[3] ··· **Assess for factors which may reduce the child's enjoyment and control of feeding.** Examples of this may be reflux and aspiration. See 'Reflux' and 'Aspiration' guidelines as relevant.

[4] ··· **Refer for radiological evaluation** to evaluate the child's swallowing function. See 'Videofluoroscopy' guidelines (pages 166–167).

[5] ··· **Use preparatory handling** to help normalize and stabilize the child's tone. Activities may include gentle rocking and use of music.

[6] ··· **Reduce environmental stimuli** so that the child can concentrate on the feeding process, and to help with the child's internal organization. It is also essential for the feeder to be able to concentrate on, and hear, the child's swallows. Reduce auditory stimuli, such as television and radio, visual stimuli such as bright lights or direct sunlight, and combined stimuli, such as the presence of extra people.

[7] ··· **Focus on normalizing sensation** in children who show hypersensitivity or desensitization. See 'Orofacial Hypersensitivity' guidelines (pages 74–77).

[8] ··· **Ensure appropriate positioning** to help with stability and increased sucking efficiency. Flexion will also help by protecting the airway. As sucking is a flexor skill, concentrate on flexion including chin tuck. Aim for an upright or semi-upright position. See 'Positioning' guidelines (pages 82–83).

[9] ··· **Focus on specific problems areas** which may be contributing to the problem: lip seal (see 'Lip Seal' guidelines, pages 61–63) and jaw instability (see 'Jaw Instability' guidelines, pages 57–58).

[10] ·· **Offer limited feeds and restricted amounts** when commencing oral feeding. Start with half a millilitre, once daily. Gradually increase the amount as the child is able to cope.

11 ·· **Thicken feeds.** Children with co-ordination problems are usually less able to cope with thin, liquid feeds as they move faster through the mouth and the child is less able to control movement of the bolus. Thickening the food offered will provide more sensory input and give the child greater control by allowing more time to organize the suck–swallow–breathe pattern, with less chance of gagging or aspirating.

▼ **Thicken the food by using a commercial thickener, baby cereal or a cornflour and water mixture.**
▼ **Make food that is less blended or add less liquid.**
▼ **Offer puréed food where liquids are currently offered.**
▼ **Always monitor the child's responses when changes are made.**

12 ·· **Stimulate and assist the swallow** directly where necessary.

▼ **Tap the tip of the tongue and the spot on the hard palate which the tip of the tongue touches (Evans-Morris and Dunn-Klein, 1987). Repeat if necessary.**
▼ **Firmly but gently, stroke a finger down the child's throat, following the floor of the mouth.**
▼ **Rub along one outer gum three times, wait for a swallow and repeat on the other outer gum.**
▼ **If a swallow is intact, Evans-Morris and Dunn-Klein (1987) recommend working on increasing its strength, length and timing.**
▼ **As the sucking rhythm emerges, use a finger or syringe to introduce carefully measured, small amounts of liquid to the outer lips, then, as appropriate, to the front of the mouth.**
▼ **Verbally remind the child to swallow where he is able consciously to achieve this, is aware of the problem and will respond to such techniques.**

13 ·· **Introduce external pacing**, where the feeder breaks the suction and defines the rhythm. This will help with internal control and the child's ability to anticipate. Pacing may only be essential during the latter part of feeding with children who present with respiratory compromise, when they are having more difficulties co-ordinating feeding.

Determine what the child is able to cope with; impose a break after two or three sucks by removing the teat, leaving the teat in place but inserting a finger into the mouth to break the suction, or tilting the bottle downwards to stop the flow of liquid (Wolf and Glass, 1992).

If external pacing is not possible, remove the teat after the first sign of respiratory difficulty to help the child learn to co-ordinate the pattern himself.

Offer slight resistance by gently tugging the bottle during sucking bursts.

The feeder should regularly test the child's self-pacing by leaving the bottle in the mouth longer than normal.

14 ·· **Slow the rate of liquid flow.**

▼ Thicken the feed, as in (11).
▼ Use external pacing, as in (13).
▼ Feed the child with the bottle at an angle.
▼ Use a slow-flow teat.
▼ Use an orthodontic teat where the hole faces upwards, rather than directing the liquid straight to the back of the mouth.
▼ Use a hard teat, as a soft teat may give too rapid a rate of flow. This will also give the child more sensory feedback. Remember, however, that a child may get more tired when sucking on a hard rather than a soft teat.

15 ·· **Facilitate improved co-ordination** directly. Apply gentle pressure to the cheeks and squeeze gently during feeding. Monitor the child's responses, as this technique can create a faster flow.

16 ·· Where appropriate, **develop breathing and vocal skills**, using blowing activities with bubbles, pinwheels, candles, straws and so on, singing, extended vocalizations and sound play, such as imitation of animal and environmental sounds.

17 ·· **Allow for maturation.** With preterm infants who evidence significant respiratory and sucking problems, oral feeding may be currently contraindicated. Focus on tube feeding, desensitization and development of non-nutritive sucking.

Initiation of the suck overview

Effects

A hungry baby will become increasingly frustrated if he is not able to initiate sucking, which in turn may lead to short-term fussing behaviours and long-term aversive behaviours. These children may tend to 'tune out' of the feeding process and may in turn be described as 'lazy' eaters.

Causes and Contributory Factors

Poor initiation of the suck may be caused by a number of reasons, including inability to inhibit the rooting reflex and start sucking, extreme mouth opening on presentation of the teat, inability to close the mouth to initiate sucking (hypertonic patterns) and excessive tongue protrusion. Where initiation of the suck was previously normal, the clinician needs to consider possible reasons, such as deterioration in respiratory status or the presence of degenerative conditions.

Normal Development

With breast-fed babies, there is a wider jaw excursion which means that it takes longer to initiate nutritive sucking. Before 33 weeks' gestation or below

131

3lb/1·4 kg in weight, the child has not reached the developmental stage where sucking and swallowing can support feeding. For a more detailed description of the development of the suck, see 'Co-ordination of the Suck–Swallow–Breathe Pattern Overview' above.

Therapy guidelines

1 ··· **Establish whether the suck reflex is present.** This usually lasts from four to six months of age. If it is consistently absent, it may indicate a depressed neurological status.

2 ··· If the child has not reached the appropriate developmental stage for sucking, focus on **oro-motor skills, desensitization and reducing hypertonicity or hypotonicity**. See 'Orofacial Guidelines', pages 74–77.

3 ··· Where a child is not getting nutrition orally and sucking may not be a part of the treatment programme, **focus on non-nutritive sucking**, particularly where the mother can breast-feed for this (use nipple shields). While the child may not be deriving nutrition via this means, he will be obtaining pleasurable oral experiences, and the mother will gain opportunities to bond. Also use dummies/pacifiers and fingers.

4 ··· **Treat the underlying problem.** If poor state and organizational abilities contribute to poor initiation of the suck, see 'Child Preparation' guidelines (pages 92–94). Other target areas may include lip seal, tongue retraction and stability.

5 ··· For all children, **reduce environmental stimuli** present so that the child can concentrate on sucking. Avoid auditory stimuli, such as televisions, visual stimuli, such as bright sunlight, and combined stimuli, such as the presence of extra people in the room.

6 ··· **Promote appropriate positioning and posturing.** As sucking is a flexor skill, encourage flexion, including chin tuck. Circular dabbing around the outside of the lips will help forward posturing for the suck. Put liquid around the outside of the lips.

7 ··· **Facilitate initiation of the suck** directly. Provide a quick stretch over the cheeks or lips.

8 ··· If the child is relatively old, for example more than one year, **focus on more advanced oro-motor skills** such as chewing, rather than sucking. See 'Chewing' guidelines (pages 30–32).

9 ··· **Control excessive rooting.** Provide firm stabilization and control of the head through appropriate positioning. Stabilize the front of the head, with jaw control if necessary. Place the teat firmly in the midline of the tongue, with slight downward pressure to give a central point of

10 ·· **Assist with mouth closure** if this is a problem. Use firm jaw control to help in physically closing the mouth, as well as grading subsequent mouth opening. Experiment with a longer teat, as a short teat may not provide sufficient sensory input to encourage mouth closure. Vibration may aid in decreasing jaw tension and support mouth closure (Wolf and Glass, 1992). This can be provided by a commercial vibrator or rapid movements of the fingers. See 'Lip Seal' guidelines (pages 61–63).

11 ·· **Encourage spontaneous mouth opening** where this is a problem. Make sure that the teat is large enough to stimulate an opening response. Mouth opening is an essential part of the rooting reflex, therefore eliciting this reflex may prompt the mouth to open (Wolf and Glass, 1992). Stimulate the lower lip by putting one or two drops of liquid on to it. Alternatively, wet a finger and rub the lower lip.

12 ·· Tongue contact with a **large, hard, wide-based teat** may stimulate the sucking burst. Try out different teats to see which one the individual child responds best to: a wide teat may depress tongue movement; a hard teat may cause the child to tire out; a soft teat may cause too rapid a rate of flow; a short teat may not provide sufficient stimulus for mouth closure.

13 ·· Gradually **introduce small amounts of liquid**. Put the liquid on the feeder's finger (or the child's) and moisten (or facilitate moistening) around the lips. This should help initiate the suck. As soon as posturing develops, put the liquid on the lower lip using a finger, spoon or syringe (which will help to measure the amount accurately), cheesecloth dipped in formula or a cotton swab. As the child develops tolerance and sucking abilities improve, increase the amounts offered. Then introduce small amounts through a teat.

Suckle to suckle overview

Function

Suckling is characterized by rhythmical in–out (forwards–backwards) tongue movements, with minimal lip and cheek involvement and large up–down jaw movements. Sucking is distinguished by a vertical, up–down pattern of tongue movement and the lips and cheeks are intimately involved in the process of feeding.

Causes of Delayed Suck Development and Contributory Factors

Problems in this area may be caused by delayed development, limiting patterns affecting the jaw, tongue, lips and cheeks, and abnormal motor patterns and reduced stability.

Normal Development

Sucking develops at age six to nine months as increased internal stability and control of the tongue, lips and so on develop. With cup drinking, suckling continues for a while to be the main form of liquid retrieval. The immature suck is usually a pattern of three to five sucks per burst, followed by a swallow. In the transitional phase, the child can have anywhere from three to 30 sucks per burst. The mature pattern is usually around ten to 30 sucks per burst, followed by a swallow.

Therapy guidelines

1 ··· **Establish** whether the child has reached the appropriate **developmental age** for sucking to have developed.

2 ··· Observe oral functions and limiting movements and concentrate on **the specific problem area**. For example, if lip seal is hindering the appropriate development of the sucking pattern, see 'Lip Seal' guidelines (pages 61–63).

3 ··· **Provide appropriate positioning.** Head and neck extension will limit sucking efficiency and affect intake. Position the child to decrease hyperextension, where appropriate (ensure that the child does not depend on neck hyperextension to maintain an airway). Focus on flexion, as sucking is a flexor skill.

4 ··· Use strategies to **reduce tongue protrusion**. See 'Tongue Protrusion/Thrust' guidelines (pages 151–153).

5 ··· **Facilitate an up–down pattern.** Assist with jaw control. Place your thumb on the child's chin bone and the rest of your hand under the jaw, and move the jaw in an up-down pattern. Tap the tongue at the point where it comes into contact with the hard palate when it is elevated for swallowing. Then tap the point of the hard palate which the tongue touches. Repeat.

6 ··· **Prevent a suckle pattern.** Place pressure on the front of the tongue, using a cup, teat or spoon placed firmly but gently on the front of tongue and lower lip. Press down and release in simulation of a suck. Do this before every suck burst.

7 ··· **Try different shaped and different sized utensils:** a long teat may encourage a suckling pattern; a wide teat may prevent thrust but restrict up–down tongue movement.

Weak suck overview

A weak or absent suck results in inefficient feeding as the child tires easily and intake is insufficient. It may be that the child starts feeding with a strong suck but that this diminishes as feeding progresses. Although there is essentially nothing wrong with the individual structures and organization of the suck, it is primarily too weak to generate continuing pressure, suction and therefore flow of liquid. There is the potential for development of aversive behaviours because of the effort involved and where hunger is not satiated.

Causes and Contributory Factors

The following is based on Wolf and Glass's (1992) discussion. They say that a weak suck can result from a number of conditions, including hypotonia and weakness (for example, Down's syndrome, myopathies), immature muscular development, as in prematurity, reduced endurance, neurological deficits, as in cerebral palsy, and respiratory problems. It can be contributed to by specific conditions: palatal clefts, a large tongue, hemangiomas and micrognathia.

Therapy guidelines

1 ··· **Consider the child's gestational age.** Children younger than 33 weeks' gestation are not yet developmentally prepared for sucking. Most feeding therapists would agree that nutritive sucking before 35 weeks places too big a demand on the child's system.

2 ··· **Examine the child for abnormal oral structures or functions** which may be affecting the strength and efficiency of the suck.

3 ··· **Focus on respiratory or endurance problems**, where these are present. See 'Respiratory Compromise' guidelines (pages 114–115) and 'Reduced Endurance' guidelines (pages 99–101).

4 ··· **Reduce environmental stimuli** so that the child can concentrate on sucking. Remove auditory stimuli, for example by turning off the television; reduce visual stimuli, such as direct sunlight or bright room lights; remove combined stimuli such as the presence of extra people in the room. Reintroduce stimuli gradually, as the child develops control and skills.

5 ··· Premature babies or physically disabled children may be in extensor patterns. As sucking is a flexor skill, **encourage correct positioning**: promote the slightly upright position, with chin tucked in (neck elongation), shoulders and hips forward; the head, neck and trunk should be symmetrical and aligned.

6 ⋯ **Normalize tone.** Focus on orofacial areas and the whole body. See 'Orofacial Hypertonia' guidelines (pages 78–79) or 'Orofacial Hypotonia' guidelines (pages 79–81), as relevant.

7 ⋯ **Focus on developing the suck outside of feeding.** Use activities such as non-nutritive sucking, using the feeder's finger, the child's finger, a dummy or a teat blocked with moistened gauze (to prevent air being swallowed). Encourage mouthing activities using relatively large rubber toys with appendages, fingers, dummies and so on.

8 ⋯ **Provide oral stability**, which may allow oral structures to produce a stronger suck, using appropriate, flexed positioning, and direct, external cheek and jaw support. Wolf and Glass (1992) recommend the use of a small bottle which may enable the feeder to use the hands and fingers for both supporting and feeding.

9 ⋯ **Encourage lip posturing and activity.** Provide circular tapping around the lips before a suck burst.

10 ⋯ **Provide slight traction.** Gently pull the teat out of the mouth to promote stronger sucking (Evans-Morris and Dunn-Klein, 1987).

11 ⋯ **Increasing the size of the bolus or amount of liquid flow** can stimulate a stronger suck. For liquids, use a medium or fast-flow teat; enlarge the hole in an ordinary teat (Warner, 1981); use thinner liquids (*ibid*). Ensure that the child is able to co-ordinate the sucking, swallowing and breathing with thinner liquids.

When using this strategy, monitor the child's response carefully. Watch for indicators that signal reduced endurance, respiratory problems, increasing incidents of choking and so on.

12 ⋯ **Use a wide-base, firm teat** for contact stimulation. With children who present with reduced endurance, remember that a firm teat may cause the child to tire more easily.

13 ⋯ With an older child, and where developmentally appropriate, **focus on more advanced patterns** such as chewing. See 'Chewing' guidelines (pages 30–32).

14 ⋯ **Ensure that nutritional requirements are being met.** Monitor weight gain through the health visitor or paediatric dietician. Where appropriate, increase the fat content of the diet. See 'Increasing Nutritional Intake' guidelines (pages 72–73). Consult the child's paediatric dietician about using assessment and the use of supplements.

Overview

Initiation of the swallow is dependent on sensory feedback from a number of areas. The most important of these are the posterior tongue, faucal arches, uvula and oropharynx. When the swallow is delayed, food can pool in the sacs (valleculae) behind the mouth. There is increased risk of choking, gagging and aspiration. Children with a delayed swallow reflex take longer than is usually observed to swallow food completely and may make many attempts to clear the food residue before they are successful.

Swallowing Stages

Swallowing has been divided into three stages, as outlined by Ray *et al* (1983), summarized here as: (1) conscious and voluntary transport of saliva and the bolus to the posterior of the oral cavity; (2) conscious and involuntary transport of saliva and the bolus through the laryngeal portion of the pharynx; and (3) unconscious and involuntary transport of saliva and the bolus through the oesophagus.

Causes and Contributory Factors

Children who have a history of oro- and nasogastric tube feeding may have become desensitized in the oropharyngeal area, with a decreased gag reflex. These children are not sufficiently sensitized to food in the posterior portion of the oral cavity, and there is the increased risk of not achieving closure of the larynx, and therefore the increased potential for choking and aspiration. Exaggerated reactions to the bolus, resulting from orofacial hypersensitivity, can cause reduced co-ordination, hypersensitive gag reflex and so on. This is seen in children with unstable neurological states.

Orofacial hypotonia can delay the child's response to sensory input. Limiting oral patterns, for example lack of tongue-tip elevation, may contribute to a delayed swallow. Other children at risk include those with respiratory compromise (Wolf and Glass, 1992). Specific congenital defects may also contribute to this problem (*ibid*).

137

Grading and Checklist

Swallowing function can be difficult to evaluate. Reilly *et al* (1995) in their study noted that the discrete oro-motor behaviours that occurred during swallowing were most difficult to record accurately. Use of the following checklist may help in determining the presence and effectiveness of the swallow. If the swallow is affected, the clinician will be able to evaluate the contributing factors. The first part of the checklist is based on the indications of swallowing dysfunction noted by Wolf and Glass (1992), with some additions.

When observing and assessing the swallow, ensure that the environment is quiet to enable the clinician to listen to and observe the child and swallow with minimal distractions. Use of the probes should help to determine the presence, timing and strength of swallowing. Individual probes will give different information in addition to focusing on the swallow. Comments should be made on movement, number of movements, timing, co-ordination and strength. With probe 1, the hyoid should move up and down in time with a swallow. This technique usually works best with children whose swallows are fairly intact, but, even if movement is felt, the co-ordination and timing of the swallow or swallows will provide valuable information.

With probe 2, as the tongue is intimately involved in the swallowing process, it should be felt to rise and fall in time with a swallow. Lack of movement in this area will help in diagnosis and treatment.

With probe 3, evaluating the gag reflex will give an indication of the child's sensitivity. Sensation in the oropharyngeal area helps the child anticipate and control the swallow. Remember that, in young infants, a gag will be naturally and normally elicited further forward than in older children.

Swallowing function can also be graded into levels of difficulty based on a number of classifications: contribution to associated problems, such as chest infections and aspiration; effect on the feeding process, specifically its length and any disruption; effect on nutritional intake and weight gain; ability to handle food consistencies; extent of oro-motor dysfunction(s) such as unco-ordination and tongue movement; laryngeal activity, such as coughing and choking; and the child's response to feeding. When grading against these guidelines, it is important to remember that other factors, such as aspiration, reflux or respiratory compromise, may be affecting feeding. The clinician must take this into account when grading, and grade with reference to the swallow function only.

To be useful, grading must be constant when applied to an individual child (that is, with a consistent clinician with consistent and interpretable classifications). Where teams are involved, the team members must agree on the classifications. Grading is only useful in these circumstances, and for evaluating the effect of therapeutic management.

GRADING	
Normal **Grade 0 swallow**	• *No dysfunction evident*
Mild **Grade 1 swallow**	• *No significant history of aspiration or chest infections* • *No significant impact on feeding, nutritional intake, or child's attitude to feeding* • *Minimal oro-motor problems* • *Infrequent coughing*
Moderate **Grade 2 swallow**	• *Occasional chest infections and indications of aspiration* • *Feeding process disrupted regularly, but not to significant degree, as child continues; feeding takes slightly longer than normal* • *Nutritional intake and weight gain below normal but extra supplements not required* • *Child evidences difficulties on swallow with thin liquids only* • *Oro-motor difficulties present and affecting swallow* • *Child coughs or chokes on regular but not consistent basis* • *Child shows some negative responses to feeding*
Severe **Grade 3 swallow**	• *Frequent chest infections with bouts of pneumonia; aspiration clinically evident* • *Feeding process significantly disrupted and oral feeding difficult* • *Nutritional intake and weight gain significantly compromised; child requires supplements or tube feeding top-up* • *Significant oro-motor difficulties present, affecting swallow* • *Coughing, choking and gagging consistent and frequent features of feeding* • *Child displays aversive behaviours to oral feeding which affect the process*
Profound **Grade 4 swallow**	• *Oral feeding contraindicated* • *Persistent chest infections, pneumonia and significant aspiration* • *Feeding process ineffective because of swallowing dysfunction, in terms of effort expended for weight gained* • *Constant choking or gagging response to oral feed* • *Child refuses oral feed*

139

SWALLOWING FUNCTION CHECKLIST

NAME		DATE

Part 1: *Clinical Observations*

FEATURES	PRESENT	ABSENT
LARYNGEAL Coughing or choking Noisy, wet upper airway sounds after individual swallows Increased noisiness over the course of feeding		
RESPIRATORY Apnoea during swallowing History of bouts of pneumonia History of chest infections		
ORO-MOTOR FUNCTIONS Inability to handle oral secretions (saliva) Multiple swallows to clear a single bolus Restricted tongue movement (specifically lack of elevation) which does not seal the oral cavity Reduced lip seal, which does not seal the oral cavity		
NUTRITIONAL Reduced or minimal intake Improved control with thicker consistencies		
SENSATIONS Reduced sensitivity, particularly in the oropharyngeal area		
ASSOCIATED CONDITIONS History or clinical signs of aspiration		
RADIOLOGY Results of swallow function based on videofluoroscopy observations		

Part 2: *Clinical Probes*

PROBES	COMMENTS
1 ···Place hand gently around the area of the hyoid bone as the child swallows	
2 ··· Place hands under the chin, where the floor of the mouth and the root of the tongue meet, as the child swallows	
3 ···Move a spatula or finger slowly back along the midline of the tongue and observe at what point the gag is elicited	

Part 3: *Summary Observations*

QUESTION	ANSWER
Is a swallow reflex present?	
Is the swallow co-ordinated with sucking and breathing?	
If a swallowing dysfunction is present, what grade/level is it?	
Are any oral dysfunctions causing or contributing to the swallowing dysfunction? If so, specify.	
Is the swallowing dysfunction so severe that oral feeding is currently contraindicated?	

▼

Therapy guidelines

1 ··· **Refer for videofluoroscopy** to confirm the presence of a swallowing dysfunction, to examine the exact nature and the contributory factors, and to help determine the course of management. See 'Videofluoroscopy' guidelines (pages 166–167).

2 ··· Where oral feeding is contraindicated, and where oral feeding is being implemented or continuing, **work on normalizing sensation and tone**. When working on desensitization begin at the level where the child is comfortable and has more control. This can be the oral level or you may need to start at his feet! Move at the child's pace, with the aim of desensitizing the area of the posterior tongue, faucal arches and so on. Use firm but gentle stroking movements towards the face.

When working at the oral level, use a plastic spatula, finger or wet cotton swab and, firmly but gently, make small movements down the centre of the tongue until just before the gag is elicited or the tongue humps. Repeat this technique when the child is ready. The point at which the gag is elicited should gradually move further back. See 'Orofacial Hypersensitivity/Desensitization' guidelines (pages 74–77) for further details. See 'Orofacial Hypertonia' guidelines (pages 78–79) or 'Orofacial Hypotonia' guidelines (pages 79–81), where relevant.

3 ··· **Reduce environmental stimuli;** this will help the child to concentrate on feeding. Remove auditory stimuli, such as the television or washing machine. Reduce visual stimuli, such as direct sunlight or bright room lights. Remove combined stimuli, such as the presence of extra people. There should be graded reintroduction of stimuli when the child has more control over swallowing.

4 ··· **Provide optimal positioning** in order to facilitate swallowing. The emphasis should be on flexion with chin tuck (neck elongation), symmetry and so on. Consult the child's paediatric occupational therapist or physiotherapist for specific and individual advice.

5 ··· **Provide cold stimulation,** recommended by a number of authorities (Evans-Morris and Dunn-Klein, 1987; Wolf and Glass, 1992), to help strengthen and trigger a faster swallow. With a child who is tube-fed, the speed of swallowing reflex may be increased by sucking on a frozen dummy/pacifier. Wolf and Glass (1992) recommend filling and freezing several at a time, because of melting. Similarly, use a cotton swab (dipped in water and frozen), an ice straw stick (water frozen in a straw and the plastic then removed) or a cold finger placed on the faucal arches. When using a straw, slip only an inch out of the tube at a time, as this will then provide the grip. Do this four or five times a day for around five minutes. Be watchful with children who have a tonic bite reflex.

Try feeding fridge-cold food at the appropriate consistency. If the child resists chilled foods, attempt gradual introduction. Chilled fruit slices can also be used. Sour, citrus tastes are a particularly good way of stimulating a swallow.

6 · · · **Stimulate and assist the swallow** directly:

▼ **Tap the tip of the tongue and the spot on the hard palate which the tip of the tongue touches (Warner, 1981). Repeat if necessary.**
▼ **Firmly but gently, stroke a finger down the child's throat following the floor of the mouth.**
▼ **Rub the outer gum with sweeping swiping movements three times and wait for the swallow. Repeat on the other side.**
▼ **Verbally remind the child to swallow if he has conscious control, can respond to this type of strategy and is aware of the problem.**

7 · · · **Introduce external pacing** where the feeder breaks the suction and defines the rhythm. Pacing may only be essential during the latter part of feeding when the child is having more difficulties co-ordinating. Providing a rhythm will allow for anticipation and organization of the swallow.

If specific difficulties are present with regard to tongue control and bolus formation, introduce a rhythm using single boluses, such as a single suck, or one spoon. When starting oral feeding, use an unattached teat, dummy or syringe, and drip small amounts of fluid into the oral cavity to provide the single bolus.

Impose a break after two or three sucks by removing the teat; leaving the teat in place but inserting a finger into the mouth to break the suction; tilting the bottle to stop the flow of liquid (Wolf and Glass, 1992).

Remove the teat after the first sign of respiratory difficulty to help the child learn to co-ordinate the suck–swallow–breathe pattern for himself.

The feeder should regularly test the child's self-pacing by leaving the bottle in the mouth longer than normal.

8 · · · For the child who is already feeding orally but having difficulties, Wolf and Glass (1992) recommend **reduction of the bolus size** now offered.

9 · · · For children with difficulties in the oral preparatory phase, **thickening the food** may help with control of the bolus as it is a more solid mass

143

and moves more slowly through the oral cavity. Additionally, the food will not spill as easily into the larynx.

Thickening can be achieved with commercial thickeners, reduced blending of home-cooked food, addition of mashed potato or baby cereal and, with liquids, by adding a cornflour and water mixture.

Be careful with cups and trainer cups, as the liquid flow may be too rapid for children with swallowing difficulties.

If developmentally appropriate, continue with fluids via the tube, cut out oral fluids and give the child semisolids or solids orally.

10 · · **Use a firm, slow-flow or medium-flow teat.** Too soft a teat will lead to the faster flow of fluid and less sensory feedback which in turn may lead to limiting motor patterns such as neck hyperextension or body arching.

11 · · **Use of specific tastes** may make swallowing easier: sweet foods can help saliva production and chewing, while sour-tasting, citrus flavours can stimulate an easier swallow. If using this strategy with an individual child, experiment first, monitoring the child's responses, particularly with regard to coping, taste preferences and hypersensitivity.

12 · · Evans-Morris and Dunn-Klein (1987) recommend a **focus on tongue-tip elevation**, given its importance in swallowing. See 'Tongue Retraction/Reduced Tongue-tip Elevation' guidelines (page 154).

13 · · **Treatment of respiratory disease** may help swallowing potential. Liaise with relevant medical staff. Where appropriate, focus on developing breathing and phonation. See 'Respiratory Compromise' guidelines (pages 114–115).

Introduction

The following checklist can help the clinician identify the function and effectiveness of the tongue in feeding. She does this mainly through observation of the tongue at rest and during feeding. Reilly et al (1995) point out that tongue movements, along with swallowing function, proved most difficult to rate in their study and this must be borne in mind when assessing tongue function.

The checklist is divided into five to enable the clinician to more easily identify the particular problem area. The section on tongue thrust is partly based on Winstock's (1994) identification of the characteristics of a tongue thrust pattern.

For a child to present with a particular difficulty, not all criteria in the section need necessarily be met. For example, a child may lack central grooving of the tongue, affecting co-ordination of the swallow and bolus control, but may not necessarily show signs of aspiration. There are always degrees of severity which have different impacts. Nutritional intake will be reduced if any particular problem is severe enough.

145

TONGUE FUNCTION CHECKLIST

NAME		DATE

Part 1: *Clinical Observations*

CHARACTERISTICS	PRESENT	ABSENT
LACK OF CENTRAL GROOVING • Tongue retracted/tight/bunched in association with hypertonia • Tongue retracted/protruded in association with hypotonia • Tongue does not groove on presentation of teat/spoon • Teat/spoon unstable • Bolus movement unco-ordinated • Choking, coughing, gagging • Aspiration present		
EXCESSIVE TONGUE-TIP ELEVATION • Tongue-tip elevates and remains elevated on presentation of teat/spoon • Teat/spoon unstable • Sucking inefficient • Intake reduced • Internal stability reduced		
TONGUE PROTRUSION • Tongue protrudes at rest • Decreased suck • Lip seal reduced • Tongue movement reduced • Hypotonia/weakness present • Saliva control reduced		
TONGUE THRUST • Thick and bunched tongue • Co-ordination of structures and bolus poor • Internal stability reduced • Jaw movement often wide • Hypertonia present • Associated with extension • Movement not rhythmical • Often starts suddenly		

TONGUE RETRACTION		
• Tongue rests further back than normal • Tongue retracts on presentation of teat/spoon • Sucking efficiency decreased • Nutritional intake reduced • Hypertonia and neck hyperextension present • Hypotonia present • Hypersensitivity present • Micrognathia present • Breathing compromised by severe retraction		

Part 2: *Summary Observations*

QUESTION	ANSWER
Is there a problem with the function and/or structure of the tongue?	
What is the particular area of difficulty?	
How does tongue function affect feeding?	

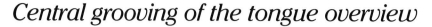

Central grooving of the tongue overview

Functions

The central groove provides a channel for liquid to travel to the pharyngeal area. It also functions to stabilize the teat and hold the bolus until swallowing is initiated. Lack of central grooving can affect co-ordination and movement of the bolus, causing it to spill over, both in the oral preparatory phase and in the pharyngeal phase. This can lead to aspiration.

Classification

Lack of central grooving of the tongue can be identified as either passive or active.

Causes and Contributory Factors

Lack of central grooving can be associated with poorly co-ordinated tongue movement and difficulty producing negative pressure suction (Wolf and Glass, 1992). Active lack of central grooving is noticed in a hypertonic (retracted, tight or bunched) tongue. Passive lack of central grooving can be observed in a hypotonic (retracted, protruded or floppy) tongue.

Therapy guidelines

1 ··· **Treat the primary problem.** For example, if retraction is an obvious problem, see 'Tongue Retraction' guidelines (page 154) in addition to those activities outlined below.

2 ··· **Position** the child to promote stability and provide support. Emphasize flexion. See 'Positioning' guidelines (pages 82–83).

3 ··· **Provide preparatory handling** to decrease or increase tone as appropriate.

▼ **Activities may include gentle rocking, bouncing.**
▼ **Use music.**
▼ **General activities such as massage may be used where appropriate.**
▼ **Consult the child's paediatric occupational therapist or physiotherapist for specific guidance.**
▼ **See 'Orofacial Hypersensitivity/Desensitization' guidelines (pages 74–77).**

4 ··· **Increase tone and sensory input of tongue.** Provide tactile input before (with a finger) feeding and during (with a teat) feeding to facilitate a groove. Wolf and Glass (1992) recommend downward pressure to the midline of the tongue; slight stroking forwards along with downwards pressure; or use of a firm, straight, narrow teat.

5 ··· Help **initiate the correct sucking pattern**. Stroke forwards and down along the midline of the tongue with the finger just before feeding. Apply the same technique with the teat before suck bursts.

Excessive tongue-tip elevation overview

Functions

When the tongue-tip is firmly and consistently elevated against the hard palate, behind the alveolar ridge, teat insertion and efficient sucking are difficult to achieve. The child may appear to be sucking, but, because the teat is under the tongue, no compression is achieved to express liquid, and intake is minimal.

Causes and Contributory Factors

Excessive tongue-tip elevation may be seen in two main areas: in premature babies, particularly when they are beginning to feed orally, and as a strategy to achieve internal stability, where that stability is reduced.

Cautionary Note

Evaluating tongue-tip movements can be difficult. As Reilly *et al* (1995) point out, this is because the lips tend to be closed during feeding. Often the clinician is best advised to watch the bottle to monitor intake. If the child is constantly elevating the tongue-tip, this will affect the amount of liquid the child is retrieving and how speedily he does so. Additionally, the clinician can *feel*, when the teat is inserted, whether the child has achieved appropriate placement and function of the tongue.

Therapy guidelines

1 ··· **Provide preparatory handling techniques** to normalize overall tone: gentle, rhythmical rocking with hypertonic children; firmer, rhythmical, more rapid rocking and carrying (for example, up and down stairs) with hypotonic children. Use calming music with hypertonic children; music with an identifiable beat and rhythm with hypotonic children. Place the child prone over the feeder's lap before feeding: this will help with flexion and more appropriate tongue placement (Evans-Morris and Dunn-Klein, 1987).

For specific and individual advice, consult the child's paediatric occupational therapist or paediatric physiotherapist.

2 ··· **Provide a stable feeding position.** Focus on encouraging neck elongation and chin tuck (forward head flexion). Provide external support through appropriate seating and/or feeder support. Consult the child's paediatric occupational therapist or paediatric physiotherapist.

149

3 ⋯ **Facilitate appropriate tongue movement** to help bring the tongue down into a more suitable position for feeding. Wolf and Glass (1992) recommend quick sweeping movements or vibration to the tongue-tip, followed by downward pressure on to the tongue. Use the prone lap position noted above before feeding.

4 ⋯ **Encourage mouth opening** which may facilitate movement of the tongue-tip into a more appropriate position. Stimulation to the lips and slight downward pressure on the jaw will help with this (Wolf and Glass, 1992). This technique can be used before teat placement, or during feeding if the tongue re-elevates. See 'Lack of Spontaneous Mouth Opening' guidelines (pages 64–65) for specific details.

5 ⋯ **Ensure appropriate teat/spoon placement.** Confirm that the teat or spoon is placed over the tongue when positioning it. Alternatively, introduce the teat to the side of the mouth, gradually working it between the gums and over the tongue.

6 ⋯ **Use an appropriate teat or spoon:** use a wide-based (for example, orthodontic) teat or spoon to help depress tongue movement; use a hard (for example, silicone) teat to provide stimulus for appropriate placement.

7 ⋯ Frequent, rhythmical bubbles should be seen if the child is sucking effectively. If the teat is placed over the tongue, but the child collapses and squashes it between the tongue and hard palate, consideration should be given to the **use of a wide-necked bottle**, with a silicone, regular shaped teat.

8 ⋯ **Ensure that adequate nutritional intake** is being received. Ask the health visitor or paediatric dietician to monitor the child's weight. Where appropriate, increase fat intake. See 'Increasing Nutritional Intake' guidelines (pages 72–73). Consider the use of supplements. Consult the child's paediatric dietician for assessment and advice.

Tongue protrusion/thrust overview

Classification

The tongue can be classified as passive where it protrudes during sucking beyond the oral cavity, usually sitting on the lower lip. The effects may include reduced suction, poor lip seal and reduced tongue movement.

The tongue can be described as active when the tongue thrusts, which Alexander (1987) describes as an abnormally strong, forward pushing of the tongue, which tends to be bunched and thick in contour. Tongue thrusts often occur as a compensatory movement to help with control of the bolus.

Causes and Contributory Factors

Passive tongue protrusion often results from hypotonia or weakness, or when the child tends to breathe through the oral airway, as when a cold is present. Active tongue thrust results from hypertonia, co-ordination and organization difficulties. The pattern may be exaggerated as the child attempts to latch on to the teat/spoon or to retrieve food.

Normal Development

Tongue protrusion and thrust are not necessarily abnormal unless they interfere with feeding. Protrusion can occur inconsistently, as when the child has a cold and needs to maintain an oral airway. Up to six months of age, children tend to have a habitual thrusting pattern, which may result in the teat being pushed out. More developed vertical movements occur from age six months, followed by lateral movements from age nine months (Winstock, 1994). A pattern of backward–forward tongue movement for cup drinking may normally occur up to age 18 months. Additionally, as the tongue often functions to provide internal stability, it may protrude until age 12 months to achieve this end where necessary.

Therapy guidelines

1 ··· Where there is active thrust or passive protrusion, **ensure that the child's breathing is not compromised**. Evaluate how much the child depends on tongue thrust or neck hyperextension for breathing; monitor breathing and state (for example, drowsiness or fitting) during feeding; evaluate whether the child has a current but temporary condition such as a cold, infection or pneumonia.

2 ··· **Provide preparatory handling** to reduce or increase tone. Use rocking and bouncing to normalize responses (Evans-Morris and Dunn-Klein, 1987). This technique should have a rhythm, gentle with the hypertonic child and more rapid with the hypotonic child. Play calming music with the hypertonic child, music with a definite and faster beat for the hypotonic child. Consult the child's paediatric occupational therapist or physiotherapist.

3 ··· **Work on correct positioning of the child** which should help provide stability to develop control. With tongue thrust which tends to be part of a total pattern of extension, inhibit this pattern: body and head should be symmetrical with neck elongation; hips and shoulders should be in flexion; arms and feet should be supported on a table or tray and foot rest (Winstock, 1994; Wolf and Glass, 1992).

With tongue protrusion which tends to result from weakness or hypotonia, focus on support and stability.

▼

4 ⋯ **Increase or decrease tone, and increase sensation in the tongue**
where appropriate by providing sensory input directly to the tongue.
With the hypertonic tongue, see 'Orofacial Hypersensitivity' (pages
74–77) and 'Orofacial Hypertonia' guidelines (pages 78–79). With the
hypotonic tongue, provide firm tapping (use finger, wet cotton swab
and so on) to the midline, from anterior to posterior; expand the
child's range of tastes and textures as appropriate; see 'Orofacial
Hypotonia' guidelines (pages 79–81).

5 ⋯ **Improve retraction.** Encouraging retraction of the tongue should help
with saliva control and potentially stimulate speech development.
Work on tone using the above four guidelines. Where appropriate,
exercise the tongue by placing a sticky substance, such as jam or
peanut butter (if possible, a mixed texture) under the tongue,
encouraging the child to retrieve it by using his tongue. When feeding,
press the spoon firmly down on the front and middle of his tongue.
Release slowly so that the lips are facilitated to remove the food and
the dysfunctional tongue pattern is inhibited (Winstock, 1994; Wolf
and Glass, 1992).

Wolf and Glass (1992) recommend the use of a commercial vibrator
or a fast rhythm with fingers where the root of the tongue is
connected to the floor of the mouth (under the chin behind the jaw
line). Winstock (1994) advises placing the hand under the chin and
applying firm pressure.

6 ⋯ **Facilitate lip activity** and initiation from the lips to help with lip seal
and remove focus from the tongue. Use the thumb and forefinger to
provide pressure on the cheeks during sucking. Place food on the lips
rather than into the mouth.

7 ⋯ **Facilitate an appropriate sucking/eating pattern** by placing pressure
on the tongue in the midline.

▼ **Place a finger firmly in the midline before using a teat.**
▼ **Use a firm, straight teat. A broad, flat teat may encourage thrusting
(Wolf and Glass, 1992). A small teat may be more easily pushed out.**
▼ **When spoon-feeding, use a large, flat-bowled spoon. Monitor for
effectiveness as it may also function to restrict tongue movement.**
▼ **Work on developing chewing skills, if developmentally appropriate,
as this should reduce protrusion/thrusting (Winstock, 1994).**
▼ **Where possible, stop or decrease the use of straws, dummies
and bottles, as these items will reinforce the thrust pattern
(Evans-Morris and Dunn-Klein, 1987).**
▼ **Do not scrape the spoon against the gum ridge when withdrawing.**

[8] ⋯ **Change the food consistency offered.** Liquids and smooth food will increase the tendency to protrude/thrust, as the tongue works harder to move this food backwards into the oral cavity. Use thickened, lumpy foods as appropriate.

[9] ⋯ **Try using larger spoonfuls of food** which may help to decrease necessity for thrust, but check to see whether this technique is restricting tongue movement.

[10] ⋯ **Use a wide utensil** such as a broad teat or spoon which will function to decrease the thrust by providing stability.

[11] ⋯ **Encourage concept development and body awareness:** body parts, such as the tongue and lips; location, such as back and front.

Tongue retraction/reduced tongue-tip elevation overview

With tongue retraction, the tongue-tip lies more further back than usual. The posterior portion of the tongue may be humped, and the tongue may be thick in appearance.

Effects

Because of reduced tongue–teat contact, sucking is less efficient and more non-nutritive. It may reinforce neck and head hyperextension in the hypertonic child (Alexander, 1987). Tongue retraction may be a compensatory strategy to achieve stability. Significant retraction of the tongue may function to block the airway and lead to respiratory compromise.

Classification

Active tongue retraction: as seen in orofacial hypertonia; passive tongue retraction: usually seen with orofacial hypotonia.

Causes and Contributory Factors

Common reasons for retraction include the following: active retraction is commonly seen in association with jaw thrust (Alexander, 1987); hypertonia and neck hyperextension can cause active retraction; hypotonia can contribute to more passive retraction; micrognathia; orofacial hypersensitivity, as in prematurity, where retraction may be a reaction to the presence of the teat.

Therapy guidelines

1 ··· **Position the child appropriately** to improve stability and support: focus on body alignment, semi-upright/upright positioning, neck elongation (chin tuck) and symmetry. Consult the child's paediatric occupational therapist or physiotherapist for specific advice.

2 ··· **Provide preparatory handling techniques.** With hypertonia, activities should function to reduce tone, as with the use of calm music. With hypotonia, rhythmical rocking and bouncing can build tone. Children can be put in a prone position either on the feeder's lap or on a wedge. Gravity will encourage the tongue to move forward (Evans-Morris and Dunn-Klein, 1987).

3 ··· **Change the tone of the tongue.** Beginning with the finger in midline position on the tongue, move from front to back. Positioning may be difficult on a very retracted tongue. Gently work the finger between the lateral gum ridge and then on to the top of the tongue. Shaking, tapping, stroking and vibration are useful strategies.

4 ··· **Encourage elevation and protrusion:**

▼ Stroke the hard palate from back to front along the midline. Use a wet finger, toothbrush or wet cotton swab. Pause (for 10 to 20 seconds, depending on the child) and repeat (Wolf and Glass, 1992).

▼ Place chocolate paste, jam or smooth peanut butter inside the gum ridge to encourage the child to use the tongue to taste or remove it. Move forward to place it on upper teeth, lips, and finally on a finger or spatula in front of the lips.

▼ Lollipops and icepops can also encourage moving tongue forward.

▼ During and after feeding, leave some food on the child's lips and point it out to him verbally or with visual cues, such as a mirror.

▼ Wolf and Glass (1992) recommend the use of a longer teat with bottle-fed children, as this may provide greater stimulation through greater tongue–teat contact.

▼ Alternatively, try a wide-based bottle with a stubby broad-based silicone teat (available generally). This functions to clamp the jaws open, so that the tongue is free to move in an extension–retraction pattern. However, see (6) below.

5 ··· **Change the bolus size** to encourage appropriate tongue movements, bearing in mind what is suitable for the individual child. Experiment with different sizes of bolus: too big a bolus will restrict tongue movement and may be dangerous; too small a bolus may not provide enough stimulation to encourage correct patterns.

6 ··· **Use a narrow teat or spoon.** A wide utensil will prevent the tongue from coming forward and functioning effectively.

Overview

A tracheostomy, which is a bypass of the airway's normal oral and nasal route, is performed when immediate or continuous ventilatory support is needed. The surgeon makes a cut directly into the laryngeal airway in the front of the neck. Children with a tracheostomy vary in the frequency and severity of feeding problems. A tracheostomy will not necessarily have an effect on feeding and oro-motor skill unless it is used after a period of prolonged intubation.

Therapy guidelines

If tracheostomy is used after **prolonged intubation**:

1 ··· Where appropriate, **focus on aspiration**, as a tracheostomy can affect laryngeal elevation and may lead to aspiration. See 'Aspiration' guidelines (pages 16–18) and 'Nasal Reflux' guidelines (page 109).

2 ··· Where appropriate, **focus on the co-ordination of the swallow** where this is affected. See 'Co-ordination of the Suck–Swallow–Breathe Pattern' guidelines (pages 129–131).

3 ··· If oral feeding is appropriate, **close off the tracheostomy fistula by placing a finger over the trachea** so that the child can swallow. If the child is dependent on the tracheostomy for breathing, release the finger once the swallow is complete to let him breathe.

4 ··· Where appropriate, **focus on communication and behaviour**. Children with tracheostomies may be susceptible to behavioural feeding problems (Arvedson, 1993a). See 'Behavioural and Communication' guidelines (pages 24–27).

5 ··· **Introduce pleasurable oro-tactile and oro-motor stimulation** as early as possible after surgery. See 'Orofacial Hypersensitivity' guidelines (pages 74–77).

155

Overview

Types of Tubes

Nasogastric tubes (through one nasal passage and via the oesophagus into the stomach) and orogastric tubes (through the oral cavity and via the oesophagus into the stomach) are most commonly seen with premature infants who have not reached the gestational milestone when they are developmentally ready for oral feeding (at least 33 and preferably 35 weeks' gestation to ensure their system is ready for oral feeding). They are also used as short-term supplementary feeding measures.

The gastro tube, placed surgically during a gastrostomy operation, is used in cases of long-term disability or anatomical problems where oral feeding is not meeting the child's nutritional requirements. The tube is placed directly through the abdomen and usually has a button flap to cover it. A nissen fundiplication (a wrap placed around the entry sphincter into the stomach) can be carried out at the same time, to prevent reflux of food. This procedure is not always successful, and reflux with or without the fundiplication can occur both back through the oesophagus and back through the tube.

Children who have a gastrostomy performed have usually had a naso- or orogastric tube before this form of feeding.

Primary Advantages of Tube Feeding

Tube feeding prevents dehydration; ensures nutrition; can ensure adequate nutritional intake; promotes weight gain; and removes pressure from carers to feed orally in difficult circumstances.

Primary Disadvantages of Tube Feeding

Tubes need to be replaced frequently. Sites require regular cleaning. Naso- and orogastric tubes in particular tend to be an obvious symbol of disability. The child may be reluctant to eat orally because of reduced hunger signals. The child may be reluctant to eat via the oral means as a result of the negative oral experiences resulting from tube cleaning, removal and reinsertion, and so on. The child may be desensitized because of frequent removal and reinsertion of naso- and orogastric tubes. The child may be hypersensitive or aversive in the orofacial area for the same reasons as above, and because of limited oral feeding experiences. Recent studies have indicated that tube-feeding may contribute to oro-motor delay.

156

Characteristics of Tube-fed Children

Evans-Morris and Dunn-Klein (1987) and Wolf and Glass (1992) note
the following characteristics of the tube-fed child which may affect oral
feeding: oral hypersensitivity; increased hyperextension; disorganized
suck–swallow–breathe pattern; gastro-oesophageal reflux; aspiration;
respiratory problems; limiting movements of the tongue, lips and so on.

Change of Feeding Method

The following checklist can be used by the clinician to help in the decision-
making process regarding the implementation of oral feeding in a child who
is tube-fed. The child need not meet all standards in order for oral feeding to
be commenced, on a trial or permanent basis.

The clinician is asked to refer to other relevant sections for more detailed
analysis of specific behaviours. For example, to determine whether a
swallow is present, refer to the 'Swallow' section. See also the 'Prefeeding'
checklist (pages 87–89).

CHANGES OF FEEDING METHOD CHECKLIST

NAME	DATE

Part 1: Clinical and Medical Observations

FACTORS	COMMENTS
READINESS • Gestational age • Presence of non-nutritive suck • Presence of nutritive suck • Prescncc of swallow • Presence of hypersensitivity	
SAFETY • Current medical condition(s) • Respiratory status • Neurological state, eg. fitting/fits • Presence and extent of aspiration • Presence and extent of reflux	
EFFECTIVENESS • Presence and potential impact of oro-motor dysfunction • Potential for weight gain or loss via oral route	
HISTORY • Results of previous oral feeding attempts	
LONG-TERM PROGNOSIS • Child's prognosis for life	
SOCIAL • Feeder expectations • Feeder commitment to carrying out oral feeding programme • Feeder resources for carrying out oral feeding programme	

Part 2: Summary Observations

QUESTION	ANSWER
Is the child ready for oral feeding?	
Would oral feeding be safe if it were implemented?	
Would oral feeding be effective?	
Do the child's history and prognosis support the commencement of oral feeding?	
Do feeder resources support the introduction of an oral feeding programme?	
Should oral feeding be implemented at this time?	

158

Therapy guidelines

1 ··· **Target oro-motor and tactile desensitization and normalization,** even if oral feeding is not the aim. It is essential to encourage pleasurable oral sensations and to reduce or minimize the effects of aversive stimuli. See 'Orofacial Hypersensitivity/Desensitization' guidelines (pages 74–77).

2 ··· **Provide counselling and support.** Feeders must be made aware that tube feeding may be a long-term process, and that the transition to oral feeding may be gradual, and not necessarily successful or complete.

3 ··· When introducing oral feeding, **observe the child's autonomic state and motor behaviours, and watch for changes in these,** for example through monitoring breathing, alertness or drowsiness, communication signals, signs of fitting, extension patterns and so on. Only maintain a level of oral feeding which is safe and efficient. See 'Stress Behaviours' checklist (page 20) for more detailed guidance.

4 ··· **Reduce environmental overstimulation.** Overstimulation can lead to an increase in tone and sensitivity, which may affect the child's state and organization, and therefore the feeder's attempts to feed successfully. Reduction in stimuli should contribute positively to the child's state and concentration. Remove auditory stimuli, such as televisions and washing machines, by turning them off; reduce or remove visual stimuli, such as direct sunlight or bright lights; remove combined stimuli, such as the presence of extra people. Gradually reintroduce stimuli as the child's coping skills improve.

5 ··· Give **opportunities for oral experience** before the introduction of oral feeding. This can help determine how the child copes with increased saliva production and give the child practice of oro-motor skills and sensations.

Encourage mouthing of the child's and feeder's finger, relatively large rubber toys with appendages and so on. Try to vary the range of objects available to the child to mouth to help him learn and adapt. Changes can also be made in the texture used.

Use the feeder's finger, the child's finger, a teat blocked with gauze, dummies and so on for non-nutritive sucking.

To further evaluate and develop sucking, dip a cheesecloth into the child's formula or mother's breast milk and introduce it into the child's mouth via the feeder's finger. The amount of liquid will be insufficient to cause choking or gagging, but give indications of ability to cope with food.

159

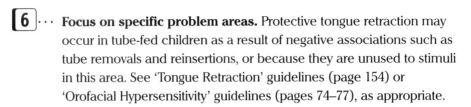

6 ··· **Focus on specific problem areas.** Protective tongue retraction may occur in tube-fed children as a result of negative associations such as tube removals and reinsertions, or because they are unused to stimuli in this area. See 'Tongue Retraction' guidelines (page 154) or 'Orofacial Hypersensitivity' guidelines (pages 74–77), as appropriate.

For co-ordination of the swallow, see 'Co-ordination of the suck–swallow–breathe pattern' guidelines (pages 129–131).

7 ··· To prepare the child for oral feeding, Evans-Morris and Dunn-Klein (1987) recommend an **increase in the range of foods given via tube** to help the child's system get used to different types of food. Check with medical staff first, as some in the medical profession do not feel that tubes are suitable for such practices. In addition, blocked tubes may lead to infection. If an attempt to increase the range of foods is undertaken, purée and dilute foods such as fruit and vegetables, or give juices.

Watch for reactions to signify the presence of allergies which may trigger feelings of discomfort or pain and encourage a negative reaction to feeding.

8 ··· Before introducing oral feeding, it is essential to help the child establish the link between hunger and oral feeding. Wolf and Glass (1992) recommend that the feeder **arrange tube-feeding so that it simulates normal hunger cycles**. When a child is fed overnight or by continuous drip, hunger sensations will be less likely to develop. Therefore instituting oral feeding will prove more difficult when there is no natural impetus or motivation to feed. The programme will be dependent on the individual child and so may vary, from three main meals with a few snacks, as with usual oral feeding, to small, more frequent meals for a younger child or infant.

9 ··· As often as possible associate tube feeds with the mouth so that the child **links the satiation of hunger with the oral area**. This may mean a predominantly oral meal topped up by tube-feeding; a limited oral snack of the appropriate consistency before tube-feeding; or pleasurable tactile stimulation of the oral area before and during feeding.

10 ·· **A combined oral feed–tube feed plan should be implemented.**
Where possible, this should simulate normal eating habits. However,
with children with reduced endurance in the initial stages of oral
feeding, or limited oral intake affecting nutrition, for example, daytime
oral feeding with overnight tube-feeding may be best, with tube-
feeding continuing to be the main source of nutrition. Tube-feeding
should be gradually eliminated from the feeding and nutrition process
where this is possible and effective. Consult the paediatric dietician to
help monitor, advise on and evaluate nutritional intake.

11 ·· **Reduce the amount of food fed via the tube to reflect the amount
given orally.** If this is not done, the child may feel overfull and
negative about oral feeding and may reject it altogether. There is also
the potential for undesirable weight gain.

12 ·· **Provide opportunities for normal socialization** at mealtimes,
whether the child is fed orally, by tube, or by a combination of the
two. The child should sit with others at mealtimes, even if the goal
is not for the child to feed at this time. He should have a plate of
food (such as finger foods, if appropriate) in front of him, to help
group bonding.

13 ·· As children who have received long-term tube-feeding may
present with behavioural problems in relation to oral feeding,
the **use of reinforcement** including appropriate praise and so on
should help progress. See 'Behaviour and Communication' guidelines
(pages 24–27).

161

Overview

Videofluoroscopy is a radiological technique whereby the child is filmed while eating. Barium is added to the child's food so that it can be seen on the screen. This procedure is useful for confirming and determining the presence and extent of anatomical and functional difficulties. It focuses mainly on the oral cavity area, but can detect reflux and aspiration which occur high up in the oesophagus and pharyngeal areas.

A barium swallow tends to examine further down the digestive tract and can indicate whether reflux or aspiration is occurring.

Reasons for Use

Use of videofluoroscopy enables the evaluation of the presence and extent of passive and unconscious processes such as reflux, aspiration and anatomical or physiological problems, and the identification of active and conscious/unconscious processes such as swallowing functions and limiting oro-motor patterns. Children with persistent behavioural feeding problems who have not been successfully weaned can also benefit from this procedure as it can demonstrate conclusively that no anatomical or functional problems exist. However, because it is a radiological technique, it should not be used without good reason.

Use of these techniques is particularly recommended where there are concerns about aspiration, reflux or swallowing function. The child must be able to swallow at least a small amount of fluid.

Radiological techniques should be used in conjunction with clinical observations. Referral for videofluoroscopy and barium swallow should not be made lightly as a radiological technique is involved. Use the 'Videofluoroscopy Referral Criteria' checklist below to determine whether an individual child should be referred. The first four sections are based on the recommended referral criteria of Arvedson and Christensen (1993) which outline behaviours and combinations of behaviours which are serious enough to warrant radiological investigation. The last section considers whether the procedure would prove effective even if warranted. Not all criteria need to be met for referral to occur.

The 'Videofluoroscopy Session' checklist will help the clinician in the structuring and evaluation of information obtained during the assessment session. For definition of food levels, see the 'Food Consistency Levels' chart (page 39).

VIDEOFLUOROSCOPY REFERRAL CRITERIA CHECKLIST

NAME		DATE
AREA	**PRESENT**	**ABSENT**
DURING FEEDING • Coughing, gagging • Excessive drooling • Increased congestion • Irritability • Lack of alertness/lethargy • Food refusal • Mealtimes lasting longer than 30 minutes		
PULMONARY STATUS • Frequent or recurrent pneumonia/ chest infections • Recurrent respiratory changes • Chronic lung changes • Infiltrates on X-ray		
GENERAL AND GASTRO INTESTINAL HEALTH • Frequent or recurrent low-grade fevers • Poor weight gain or weight loss • Emesis • Reflux		
STRUCTURAL • Suspected tracheal fistula • Vocal cord paralysis or paresis		
PRACTICAL QUESTIONS • Is the child able to take at least 5 ml orally? • Is the child's state amenable to the procedure (for example, reduced alertness or fits)? • Is the child able to sit or stand by himself or with use of equipment? • Has parental consent been received?		

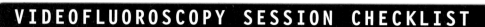

VIDEOFLUOROSCOPY SESSION CHECKLIST

NAME	DATE

ENVIRONMENT

Note people present
Note seating equipment used
Note food utensils used

POSITIONING

Note child's position (and changes to it) during feeding
Note position of feeder in relation to child

CHILD'S RESPONSES

- To general situation
- To introduction of barium/food
- To feeder
- To positioning and changes to position
- To various food textures
- Note child's general tone and tonal variations during session

AMOUNT GIVEN

- Level 1
- Level 2
- Level 3
- Level 4
- Level 5
- Level 6

- Level 7
- Level 8
- Level 9
- Level 10
- Level 11

SPEED OF BOLUS MOVEMENT

- At oral phase
- At pharyngeal phase
- At oesophageal phase

Is speed affected by consistency of food?

IF DELAYED IS IT A FUNCTION OF

- General co-ordination of the suck–swallow–breathe process?
- Problems with bolus formation?
- Delayed swallow reflex?
- Tonal abnormalities?
- Sensation abnormalities?
- Respiratory status?
- Other?

ANATOMY AND FUNCTION

Note abnormal structure, movement and function

ANATOMY	FUNCTION
• Tongue • Lips • Palate • Velopharynx • Cheeks • Jaw • Pharynx • Oropharyngeal space • Larynx • Oesophagus • Other	

PASSAGE OF BOLUS

- Does bolus clear sides of mouth and valleculae?
- Does bolus move smoothly through mouth etc?
- Is passage dependent on consistency?
- Is swallow triggered on time so that bolus passes safely?
- Are there signs of aspiration?
- Are there signs of reflux?

HYPERSENSITIVE REACTIONS

Note indications of hypersensitivity such as hyperactive gag reflex, mouth closure in response to food introduction or reactions to food being placed in the mouth.

Therapy guidelines

1 ⋯ Some radiology suites will not be designed or set up for children. **Make a preliminary visit to the suite** with the paediatric occupational therapist to familiarize yourself with the resources. This also ensures that the speech and language therapist and the paediatric occupational therapist are prepared, have the appropriate equipment to hand and can adapt positively to the circumstances, which will increase the reliability of the procedure and the results gained.

2 ⋯ **Prepare the child for the experience and the environment ahead of time.** This will involve explaining the reasons, layout and people involved in the assessment session.

3 ⋯ Try to **relax the child** both before and during the session with familiar and favourite toys, music, books, stories and so on, but making sure that the child is not so tired that feeding is affected.

4 ⋯ Where possible, **videotape the procedure**. The tape can be viewed by professionals and parents at leisure after the procedure. It can be used for more detailed analysis after the session. This is particularly relevant if the speech and language therapist is the person feeding the child during the session, as it can be difficult to view and feed at the same time. Taping can also be used as a record of progress.

5 ⋯ It is essential to perform the procedure with the child in as **upright a position as possible** or appropriate, as the usual X-ray technique of having the client lying down is inappropriate and atypical for feeding. Consult the paediatric occupational therapist about positioning.

6 ⋯ Large amounts of food are not required but, where possible and appropriate, a **range of consistencies should be used**. This includes fluids, purées and solids.

7 ⋯ **Use familiar utensils and foods.** This means that the parent will need to bring in their own equipment and home-prepared food in a range of consistencies.

8 ⋯ **Radiological techniques are not necessarily conclusive**. There may be a number of reasons for this: the child may not 'perform' on the day; the time available may not be sufficient for the child; the bolus volume given during the procedure may not reflect the quantity received at regular mealtimes, and the problems seen then may not occur during the session. By monitoring and by liaising with the paediatric dietician, the clinician should have made herself aware of the child's normal intake and taken this into consideration when estimating the results of the videofluoroscopy.

166

9 ··· **Use the 'Videofluoroscopy Session' checklist** (page 164) to help
collate and clarify information from the procedure.

REFERENCES

Alexander R, 'Prespeech and feeding development', McDonald Eugene T (ed), *Treating Cerebral Palsy: For clinicians, by clinicians,* ProEd, Austin, Texas, 1987.

Arvedson JC, 'Feeding with Craniofacial Abnormalities', Arvedson JC & Brodsky L (eds), *Paediatric Swallowing and Feeding: Assessment and Management,* Whurr Publishers, San Diego, California, 1993a.

Arvedson JC, 'Management of Swallowing Problems', Arvedson JC & Brodsky L (eds), *Paediatric Swallowing and Feeding: Assessment and Management,* Whurr Publishers, San Diego, California, 1993b.

Arvedson JC & Christensen S, 'Instrumental Evaluation', Arvedson JC & Brodsky L (eds), *Paediatric Swallowing and Feeding: Assessment and Management,* Whurr Publishers, San Diego, California, 1993.

Brodsky L, 'Drooling in Children', Arvedson, JC & Brodsky L (eds), *Paediatric Swallowing and Feeding: Assessment and Management,* Whurr Publishers, San Diego, California, 1993.

Dodds WJ, 'The physiology of swallowing', *Dysphagia* 3, pp171–178, 1989.

Dodimead L, 'The development of eating behaviour in early childhood', *The Australian Journal of Early Childhood* 13 (4), pp3–9, 1988.

Ekedahl C, Mansson I & Sanberg N, 'Swallowing dysfunction in the brain damaged with drooling', *Acta Otolaryngology* 78, pp141–149, 1978.

Evans-Morris S & Dunn-Klein M, *PreFeeding Skills,* Therapy Skills Builders, Tucson, Arizona, 1987.

Goode RL & Smith RA, 'The surgical management of sialorrhea', *Laryngology* 80, pp1078–1089, 1970.

Heidelise ALS, 'A synactive model of neonatal behavioural organisation: Framework for the assessment of neurobehavioural development in the premature infant and for support of infants and parents in the neonatal intensive care environment', Sweeney JK (ed), *The high risk neonate: Developmental therapy perspectives – physical and occupational therapy in paediatrics,* Haworth, 1986.

Neal P, 'Feeding the preterm baby', *Professional Care of the Mother and Child* 5 (6), pp1530–1555, 1995.

Palmer JB, 'Electromyography of the muscles of oropharyngeal swallowing: basic concepts', *Dysphagia* 3, pp192–198, 1989.

Ray SA, Bundy AC & Nelson DL, 'Decreasing drooling through techniques to facilitate mouth closure', *The American Journal of Occupational Therapy* 37 (11), pp749–753, 1983.

Reilly S, Skuse D, Mathisen B & Wolke D, 'The objective ratings of oral motor functions during feeding', *Dysphagia* 10, pp177–191, 1995.

Satter EM, 'Childhood eating disorders', *Journal of the American Dietetic Association* 86 (3), pp357–361, 1986.

Strawbridge-Domaracki L & Sisson LA, 'Decreasing drooling through oral motor stimulation in children with multiple disabilities', *The American Journal of Occupational Therapy* 44 (8), pp680–684, 1990.

Warner J, *Helping the Handicapped Child with Early Feeding*, Winslow Press, Bicester, Oxon, 1981, out of print.

Winstock A, *The Practical Management of Eating and Drinking Difficulties in Children*, Winslow Press, Bicester, Oxon, 1994.

Wolf LS & Glass RP, *Feeding and Swallowing Disorders in Infancy*, Therapy Skill Builders, Tucson, Arizona, 1992.

169

INDEX

Location references in *italic* indicate tables.

prefeeding organization 94, 95
reduced endurance 100
spoon feeding 123
suck, delayed development 134
suck, initiating 133
swallowing dysfunction 144
tongue protrusion 152, 153
tongue retraction 154
tongue-tip elevation, excessive 150
tonic bite reflex 53
videofluoroscopy 166
weak suck 136
schedule
cleft lip and palate 34
reduced endurance 100
stages, feeding cycles 128
time spent on 9, 25
feeds, quantity
aspiration 16-170
cup drinking 35
gastro-oesophageal reflux 107
reduced endurance 100
suck-swallow-breathe pattern problems 129
finger foods 38, 41, 55
flavours
cup drinking 35
increasing range 32
introducing new 41, 49, 76
swallowing dysfunction 144
flexed pattern, tonic bite reflex 53, 54
flexion, positioning 82, 85
food
allergies 108, 160
clearance, practices to facilitate 18
consistency 38-41
hypersensitive children 76
levels 39, 40
therapy guidelines 41
contributing to aspiration 18
diary 1, 68-9, 70, 71
play
behaviour and communication 25
chewing 32
gagging and choking 49
gastro-oesophageal reflux 108
preferences 67
refusal 19, 25, 26
temperature 32, 67
transitions 42
see also liquids to solids; tube feeding,
transition to oral feeding

173

Also Available from Winslow

The Practical Management of Eating & Drinking Difficulties in Children

April Winstock

Established as a major work of reference, this title provides information on how to help children who have difficulty in eating and drinking. The advice is applicable to cerebral palsy, Riley-Day syndrome and many other disabilities as well as to general development delay. Clearly illustrated throughout, the wealth of practical information contained in this text will make it indispensable for anyone trying to overcome feeding difficulties.

In dealing with day-to-day management of clients, the Winslow Working with ... series has established an enviable reputation as the essential resource for every speech and language professional. Some of the titles available are:

Working with
Swallowing

Judith Langley

This practical book examines in detail the structures and processes involved in eating and drinking. Every aspect is considered, from the senses of taste and smell and the value of oral hygiene to the neural organisation of chewing and swallowing, as well as the significance of breakdowns in any of the functions involved.

The reader will find a wealth of sound advice and helpful suggestions for developing individual swallowing rehabilitation programmes in addition to thorough assessment procedures.

Working with
Children's Language

Jackie Cooke & Diana Williams

Containing a wealth of ideas and a wide range of activities, the practical approach to language teaching has helped establish this book as a leading manual in its field. It includes games, activities and ideas suitable for developing specific language skills.

Working with
Children's Phonology

Gwen Lancaster & Lesley Pope

Successfully bridging the gap between theory and practice, this book provides a wealth of creative ideas for lively and entertaining activities for therapy. This thoroughly practical manual also examines recent advances in the analysis and description of phonological disorders and describes their management within the clinic.

Working with
Cleft Palate

Jackie Stengelhofen

Here is a hands-on manual full of practical ideas for therapists working with children or adults. A detailed account of principles and practice is provided, inspiring confidence for all professionals concerned with the treatment of cleft palate.

Each stage of case management, from physical assessment to intervention and treatment procedures, is explained. There is also an exploration of how the condition affects the vocal tract function, which can result in articulatory, resonatory and phonatory problems.

Working with
Dysarthrics

Sandra Robertson & Fay Thomson

This is a unique source of ideas for individual and group speech therapy with patients who have dysarthria as a result of acquired neurological damage.

Current theory on the problems of dysarthria and assessment procedures as well as the principles, goals and efficacy of treatment are discussed. These are linked with activities and large print to improve all aspects of motor speech.

Working with
Dysfluent Children
Practical Approaches to Assessment & Therapy
Trudy Stewart & Jackie Turnbull

This essential manual analyses dysfluency in children and provides the reader with practical ways of handling these difficulties in collaboration with the child, parents and carers.

Complete with case studies, key summaries, notes on teaching the easy onset technique, lists of therapy resources and a comprehensive index, this text will be an essential reference for all those involved in working with dysfluent children.

Working with
Dysphonics

Stephanie Martin

Here is an invaluable resource and reference book for speech therapists in practice as well as students in training.

The structures and processes involved in normal phonation are examined in detail and possible breakdowns at different levels are identified. Sound advice on assessment, management and specific treatment approaches is offered, following careful consideration of the case history. Recent advances in the use of instrumentation for assessment are acknowledged, but the emphasis is on traditional procedures.

Working with
Dyspraxics

Susan Huskins

This informative working manual brings together current findings on dyspraxia of speech in adults and presents a meaningful approach to its assessment, diagnosis and treatment.

The author deals lucidly with a wide range of topics – from differential diagnosis to specific therapy procedures and alternative methods of communication.

Articulatory diagrams are included; these are arranged phonetically for ease of access and may be photocopied.

Working with
Laryngectomees

Eryl Evans

This is a practical manual of positive therapy ideas and management approaches for every professional working with laryngectomy patients. It outlines involvement at all stages of rehabilitation, from pre-operative to completion, covering oesophageal voice acquisition, the use of communication aids and recent advances in surgical voice restoration.

The author considers the laryngectomee within the wider environment and thus there are plenty of suggestions for dealing with day-to-day care, spouse and family involvement as well as sources of advice and information.

Working with
Oral Cancer

Julia Appleton & Jane Machin

This latest addition to the series presents clinicians with a practical working knowledge of swallowing and speech disorders arising as a result of surgery for carcinoma of the oral cavity.

With very little written matter presently available on this specialist subject area, this title will be invaluable to therapists and students who wish to develop new skills or would like to build on existing knowledge.

These are just a few of the many therapy resources available from Winslow. A free catalogue will be sent on request. For further information please contact:

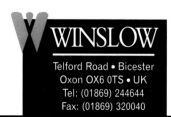

WINSLOW
Telford Road • Bicester
Oxon OX6 0TS • UK
Tel: (01869) 244644
Fax: (01869) 320040